Exam Preparatory Manual
for Undergraduates
ORTHOPEDICS

Exam Preparatory Manual for Undergraduates
ORTHOPEDICS

SECOND EDITION

Sandip Ghosh MS (Ortho) PGI (Chandigarh)
Principal
Department of Orthopedics
RG Kar Medical College and Hospital
Kolkata, West Bengal, India

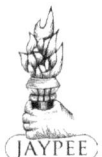

JAYPEE BROTHERS MEDICAL PUBLISHERS
The Health Sciences Publisher
New Delhi | London

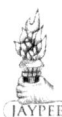

Jaypee Brothers Medical Publishers (P) Ltd

Headquarters
EMCA House
23/23-B, Ansari Road, Daryaganj
New Delhi 110 002, India
Landline: +91-11-23272143, +91-11-23272703
+91-11-23282021, +91-11-23245672
E-mail: jaypee@jaypeebrothers.com

Corporate Office
Jaypee Brothers Medical Publishers (P) Ltd.
4838/24, Ansari Road, Daryaganj
New Delhi 110 002, India
Phone: +91-11-43574357
Fax: +91-11-43574314
E-mail: jaypee@jaypeebrothers.com

Overseas Office
JP Medical Ltd.
83, Victoria Street, London
SW1H 0HW (UK)
Phone: +44-20 3170 8910
Fax: +44(0)20 3008 6180
E-mail: info@jpmedpub.com

Website: www.jaypeebrothers.com
Website: www.jaypeedigital.com

© 2021, Jaypee Brothers Medical Publishers

The views and opinions expressed in this book are solely those of the original contributor(s)/author(s) and do not necessarily represent those of editor(s) of the book.

All rights reserved by the author. No part of this publication may be reproduced, stored or transmitted in any form or by any means, electronic, mechanical, photocopying, recording or otherwise, without the prior permission in writing of the publishers.

All brand names and product names used in this book are trade names, service marks, trademarks or registered trademarks of their respective owners. The publisher is not associated with any product or vendor mentioned in this book.

Medical knowledge and practice change constantly. This book is designed to provide accurate, authoritative information about the subject matter in question. However, readers are advised to check the most current information available on procedures included and check information from the manufacturer of each product to be administered, to verify the recommended dose, formula, method and duration of administration, adverse effects and contraindications. It is the responsibility of the practitioner to take all appropriate safety precautions. Neither the publisher nor the author(s)/editor(s) assume any liability for any injury and/or damage to persons or property arising from or related to use of material in this book.

This book is sold on the understanding that the publisher is not engaged in providing professional medical services. If such advice or services are required, the services of a competent medical professional should be sought.

Every effort has been made where necessary to contact holders of copyright to obtain permission to reproduce copyright material. If any have been inadvertently overlooked, the publisher will be pleased to make the necessary arrangements at the first opportunity. The **CD/DVD-ROM** (if any) provided in the sealed envelope with this book is complimentary and free of cost. **It is Not meant for sale.**

Inquiries for bulk sales may be solicited at: jaypee@jaypeebrothers.com

Exam Preparatory Manual for Undergraduates: Orthopedics

First Edition: 2017
Second Edition: **2021**
ISBN: 978-93-5465-172-4

Dedicated to

*My parents
and my beloved sons
Suddhabrata and Subhodripto*

PREFACE TO THE SECOND EDITION

In this second edition, I have added few more X-rays, instruments and implant images. Addition of some new topics, elaborate descriptions of some topics, necessary for undergraduate MBBS students, along with few more question-answers, related to orthopedic viva-voce examination done. Correction of printing mistakes in the first edition is taken care of. Hope this book will be very helpful for undergraduate MBBS students for their Final MBBS examination, as written according to CBME course curriculum of latest NMC guidelines..

Sandip Ghosh

PREFACE TO THE FIRST EDITION

This book has been written to meet the requirement of undergraduate students getting basic ideas in orthopedics (medical science). Ever since the orthopedics section in medical science was introduced in India, a need has been felt for a book on this subject of basic standard and undergraduate (both practical and theoretical) exam-oriented. A keen attempt has been made to make the book useful and interesting and required to deal with trauma (fractures), tumor, sports medicine, congenital and metabolic disorders and related orthopedic surgery, which is required for undergraduate MBBS examination. Leaving aside all the necessary things, only the essential facts have been discussed in this book. It has a direct link with practical work that all the common and complicated troubles of orthopedics have been explained very clearly and easy to understand and easy to memorize also.

It has been experienced that students are lacking in their confidence to face long cases, short cases, instruments, implants, X-rays, viva voce and short-note type questions. Therefore, this book has been written in such a way that it may equip the students with basic knowledge to face theoretical as well as practical examination in orthopedics part of surgery examination. It is hoped that this book will be useful for all the students of MBBS and undergraduate medical students.

Sandip Ghosh

ACKNOWLEDGMENTS

I am really grateful to the authors of all standard textbook of orthopedics, from which I have enriched myself throughout my study life and also in my professional life. I am also thankful to Director (Medical Education), Department of Health and Family Welfare, West Bengal, and my colleagues and students for continuous inspiration of writing this book.

I am also grateful to my parents Mr Satyapriya Ghosh and Mrs Malaya Ghosh, for their tremendous support throughout my career.

I am specially thankful to my spouse Dr Sangeeta Ghosh, for her continuous support. I am also grateful to my loving sons Suddhabrata Ghosh and Subhodripto Ghosh, for bearing with me.

I would like to appreciate the constant support and encouragement of Shri Jitendar P Vij (Group Chairman), Mr Ankit Vij (Managing Director), Mr MS Mani (Group President), Dr Madhu Choudhary (Publishing Head-Education), Ms Pooja Bhandari (Production Head), Ms Sunita Katla (Executive Assistant to Group Chairman and Publishing Manager), Ms Samina Khan (Executive Assistant to Publishing Head-Education), Ms Seema Dogra (Cover Visualizer), Mr Rajesh Sharma (Production Coordinator), Mr Laxmidhar Padhiary (Proofreader), Ms Uma Adhikari (Typesetter) and Mr Gopal Singh Kirola (Graphic Designer) of M/s Jaypee Brothers Medical Publishers (P) Ltd., New Delhi, India.

CONTENTS

1. **Genetic Disorders**   1
   - Congenital Talipes Equinovarus   1
   - Congenital Vertical Talus   6
   - Developmental Dysplasia Hip   7
   - Osteogenesis Imperfecta   8
   - Skeletal Dysplasia   9
   - Congenital Tibial Pseudoarthrosis   12
   - Spina Bifida   12

2. **Infection**   14
   - Osteomyelitis   14
   - Septic Arthritis of Hip   17
   - Arthrotomy   18

3. **Rheumatic Disorders**   19
   - Rheumatoid Arthritis   19
   - Ankylosing Spondylitis   21
   - Other Rheumatic Disorders   22

4. **Crystal Deposition Disorder**   23
   - Gout   23

5. **Osteoarthritis**   25
   - Genu Varum   26
   - Genu Valgum or Knock Knee (Reverse of Genu Varum)   26
   - Total Knee Replacement   27

6. **Avascular Necrosis (Osteonecrosis)**   28
   - Total Hip Replacement   29
   - Osteoporosis   30

7. **Metabolic and Endocrine Disorders**   30
   - Rickets   31
   - Osteochondroma or Exostosis   35

8. **Bone Tumors**   35
   - Simple Bone Cyst   36
   - Aneurysmal Bone Cyst   37
   - Eosinophilic Granuloma   37
   - Giant Cell Tumor   38
   - Malignant Tumor of Bone   39
   - Osteosarcoma   39
   - Ewing's Sarcoma   41
   - Chondrosarcoma   41
   - Multiple Myeloma   42

9. **Amputations**   43
   - Lower Limb and Upper Limb Amputation   43
   - Ideal Amputation Stump   43
   - Indications of Amputation   44
   - Below-Knee Amputations   44
   - Syme's Amputation   45
   - Knee Injury   46
   - Hemarthrosis   46

10. **Sports Injury**   46
    - Knee Ligament Injuries   48

11. **Fractures**   50
    - Stress Fracture   50
    - Pathological Fracture   51
    - Open (Compound) Fracture   52
    - External Fixation   52
    - Green Stick Fracture   53

12. **Fractures Around Hip Joint**   54
    - Fracture Neck of Femur   54
    - Intertrochanteric Fracture   56
    - Subtrochanteric Fracture   57
    - Fracture Head of Femur   58
    - Acetabular Fracture   59
    - Fracture Pelvis   59

13. **Fracture Around Knee and Above**   61
    - Fracture Patella   61
    - Tension Band Wiring   62
    - Fracture Femoral Condyle   62
    - Tibial Plateau Fracture or Fracture of Tibial Condyle   63
    - Knee Dislocation   64
    - Fracture Shaft of Femur   65

14. **Fracture Around Ankle and Above**   67
    - Fracture of Tibia   67
    - Fracture Medial Malleoli and Fracture Lateral Malleoli   68
    - Fracture Talus   69
    - Fracture Calcaneum   70
    - Fracture Tarsal Bones   70
    - Fracture Metatarsal Bones or Fracture Phalanx   71

15. **Fracture Around Shoulder**   72
    - Fracture Clavicle   72
    - Dislocation of Shoulder   73
    - Recurrent Dislocation of Shoulder   74
    - Fracture Neck of Humerus   74
    - Fracture Shaft of Humerus   75
16. **Fracture Around Elbow Joint**   76
    - Supracondylar Fracture Humerus (Extra-articular)   76
    - Medial Condyle Fracture   78
    - Lateral Condyle Fracture   79
    - Dislocation of Elbow   80
    - Radial Head Fracture   81
    - Fracture Olecranon   82
    - Intercondylar Fracture   82
    - Cubitus Varus and Valgus   83
    - Fracture Both Bone Forearm   84
    - Monteggia Fracture Dislocation   84
    - Galeazzi Fracture Dislocation   85
17. **Fractures Around Wrist**   86
    - Colles Fracture   86
    - Fracture Metacarpals/Fracture Phalanges   87
    - Scaphoid Fracture   87
18. **Spinal Disorders**   88
    - Slipped Disk   88
    - Kyphoscoliosis   88
    - Cervical Spondylosis   90
    - Spondylolisthesis   90
19. **Short Notes**   92
    - Brodie's Abscess   92
    - Made Lung's Deformity   93
    - Radial Club Hand   93
    - Ulnar Club Hand   94
    - Bone Tumors of Cartilage Origin   94
    - Carpal Tunnel Syndrome   94
    - De Quervain's Disease   95
    - Ankylosis   95
    - Frozen Shoulder   96
    - Bone Graft   97
    - Ruptured Tendo-Achilles   98
    - Mallet Finger   98
    - Trigger Finger   99
    - Codmann's Triangle   99
    - Bone Scan   100
    - Clinical Application   100
    - Housemaid's Knee   100
    - Baker's Cyst   100
    - Arthroscopy   101
    - Tardy Ulnar Nerve Palsy/Ulnar Claw Hand   101
    - Wrist Drop   102
    - Myositis Ossificans   102
    - Tennis Elbow   103
    - Golfer's Elbow   103
    - Volkmann's Ischemic Contracture   104
    - Ganglion   104
20. **Practical Examination (Orthopedics)**   105
    - Long Cases   105
    - History Taking/Writing: in a Long Case of Hip   105
    - Nonunion Fracture Neck of Femur   107
    - Tuberculosis of Hip   109
    - Neglected Dislocation Hip   110
    - Post-septic Sequelae—Usually Occurs in Child   111
    - Chronic Osteomyelitis   112
    - Perthes Disease   113
    - Caries Spine (TB Spine)   115
21. **Short Cases**   117
    - Malunion   117
    - Nonunion   118
    - Cubitus Varus   119
    - Cubitus Valgus   120
    - Foot Drop   121
    - Wrist Drop   121
    - Ulnar Claw Hand   122
    - Genu Varum   123
    - Genu Valgum   124
22. **Operative**   125
    - K-Nail in Fracture Shaft of Femur (Fracture SOF)   125
    - Plate Fixation in Fracture Shaft of Femur   126
    - Plate Fixation in Fracture Both Bone Forearm   126
23. **Instruments**   128
    - Screw Driver   128
    - Periosteum Elevator   128
    - Bone Pliers   128
    - Bone Chisel—One End is Bevelled   129
    - Sequestrectomy Forcep—Single Hinge   129

- Bone Tap 130
- Bone Cutting Forcep—Double Hinge 130
- Bone Nibbler 131
- Bone Lever (Bristow's) 131
- Bone Lever—Pointed 131
- Allis Tissue Forceps 132
- Needle Holder 132
- Bone Curette 133
- Hemostatic Forceps 133
- Bone Gouge 133
- Osteotome 134
- Bone Holding Forcep 134
- Mallet/Hammer 134
- Rimmer 135
- Cannulated Rimmer 135
- Mannmann Electric Drill Hand Piece with Key 135
- Drill Bit 136
- Depth Gaze 136
- Drill Guide 136
- Impacter 137
- Patella Holding Forcep 137
- Langenbeck's Retractor 137
- Bone Holding Forceps 138
- Bone Awl With Hole 138
- Plate Holding Forceps 138
- Lowmanns Bone Holding Clamp 139
- T Handle for Pin Introduction 139
- Spanner Wrench for External Fixator 139
- Hand Drill with Key 140

24. **Implants** 141
- Austin Moore Prosthesis 141
- Bipolar Prosthesis 141
- Steinmann Pin (4.5 mm) 141
- Steinmann Pin with Bholer's Stirrup 142
- Cortical Screw 142
- Cancellous Screw 142
- Limited Contact Dynamic Compression Plate 143
- K-Nail 143
- K-Wire 144
- Rush Nail 144
- Philos Plate 144
- Reconstruction Plate 145
- Dynamic Hip Screw with Barrel Plate 145
- Distal Femoral Locking Plate 145
- Distractor of External Fixator with Allen Key 146
- AO Tubular Rod and Universal Clamp 146
- Schanz Pin 147
- Cortical and Cancellous Schanz Pin 147
- Cancellous Schanz Pin 147
- Cortical Schanz Pin 148
- Cortical Schanz Pin with Universal Clamp 148
- Universal Clamp with T-Clamp and Tube-Tube Clamp 148
- AO Tubular Rod with Universal Clamp 149
- K-Nail with Rimmer (Below) 149

25. **X-rays** 150
- X-ray of Fracture Both Bone Leg (Fracture Tibia Distal 1/3rd, and Fibula Upper 1/3rd) 150
- X-ray of Fracture Supracondylar Humerus in a Child 150
- X-ray of Fracture Pelvis 151
- X-ray of Fracture Shaft of Distal Femur in Child 151
- X-ray of Fracture Shaft of Femur in a child 152
- X-ray of Fracture Both Bone M/3 of Forearm in adult 152
- X-ray of Fracture Both Bone leg at M/3 and D/3 Junction 153
- X-ray of Comminuted Fracture Shaft of Distal Humerus 153
- X-ray of M/3 Fracture Clavicle 153
- X-ray of Fracture Proximal Humerus 154
- X-ray of Fracture Both Bone Forearm at M/3 to D/3 Junction 155
- X-ray of Fracture Both Bone Leg (Fracture Shaft of Lower 1/3rd of Tibia and Upper 1/3rd of Fibular Shaft) 155
- Internal Fixation with Tens in a Fracture Both Bone Forearm in Child After Closed Reduction 156
- X-ray of Fracture Acetabulum 156
- X-ray of Fracture Shaft of Femur 157
- Internal Fixation with Closed Interlocking Nail with Bolts in A Case of Fracture Shaft of Femur 157

- Internal Fixation with Herbert (Headless) Screw for Fracture Scaphoid, After Open Reduction 158
- Internal Fixation with Medial Buttress Plate after Closed Education in a Medial Condyle Fracture Tibia with K-Wire Fixation for Fracture Neck of Fibula 159
- X-ray of Fracture Both Bone Foream 159
- Internal Fixation with LCDCP for Fracture Both Bone Forearm After Open Reduction 160
- X-ray of Fracture Neck of Femur 160
- Bipolar (Prosthesis) Hemiarthroplasty in a Case of Fracture Neck of Femur, with Avascular Necrosis of Opposite Hip 161
- Bipolar (Prosthesis) Hemiarthroplasty in a Case of Fracture Neck of Femur 161
- X-ray of Fracture Intertrochanteric Femur 162
- Internal Fixation with Dynamic Hip Screw With Barrel Plate With Cotical Screw, after Closed Reduction, in a Case of Intertrochanteric Fracture 162
- Communited Fracture Calcanaum—Lateral View 163
- X-ray of Comminuted Fracture Both Bone Leg 163
- Internal Fixation with Closed Interlocking Nail in a Case of Fracture Both Bone Leg 164
- X-ray of Uniting Fracture of Both Bone Leg with Interlocking Nail in Situ 164
- X-ray of Fracture Supracondylar Humerus in a Child with Pop Back Slab 165
- X-ray Showing Fracture Patella (Both Anteroposterior and Latral View of Knee) 165
- X-ray of Fracture Distal Radius (Colles Extra-articular) 166
- X-ray of Galeazzi Fracture Dislocation (Fracture of the Distal Radius with Distal Radioulnar Joint Dislocation) 166
- Fracture Neck of Humerus with Dislocation Shoulder 167
- X-ray of Fracture Shaft of Humerus 167
- X-ray of Fracture Shaft of Tibia with Bimalleolar Fracture 168
- X-ray of Depressed Fracture Latral Condyle of Tibia 168
- X-ray of Fracture Distal Radius with Vertical Split Up to Shaft 169
- X-ray of Fracture Olecranon 169
- X-ray Aneurysmal Bone Cyst in Lower End of Tibia 170
- X-ray of Leg of a Case of Osteogenesis Imperfecta in a Child 170
- X-ray of Both Bone Leg in a Case of Osteogenesis Imperfecta 171
- X-ray of a Post-septic Sequelae of Hip 171
- X-ray of Chronic Osteomyelitis of Radius in a Child 172

Index 173

CHAPTER 1: Genetic Disorders

■ CONGENITAL TALIPES EQUINOVARUS (CTEV)

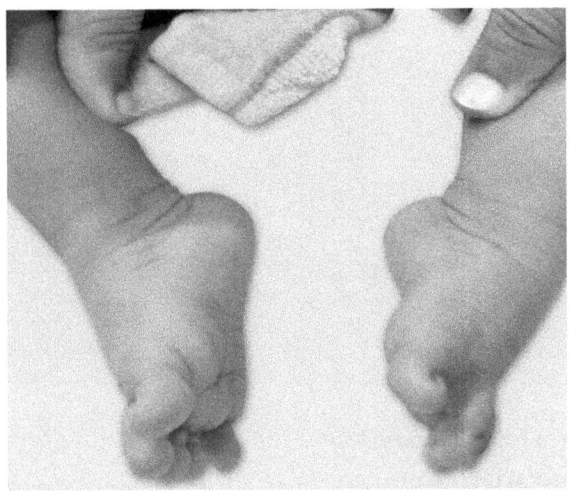

Q Why are you saying that the deformity is congenital?
- Deformity present since birth
- Bilateral presentation
- Male child (usually) affected

Q What is the meaning of talipes?

Meaning of talipes (2 school of thoughts)
- Abnormality in pes (foot)
- Abnormality in talus (Main deforming force related to talus)

Q What are the components of CTEV?
- Hindfoot—equinus
- Midfoot varus
- Forefoot adduction and supination
- Internal tibial torsion.

2 Genetic Disorders

Q How do you know equinus is present?

Hindfoot equinus confirmed by:
- Small highly placed heel, facing towards sky
- Equinus crease at posterior aspect of heel
- Tight TA (tendo-Achilles tendon)

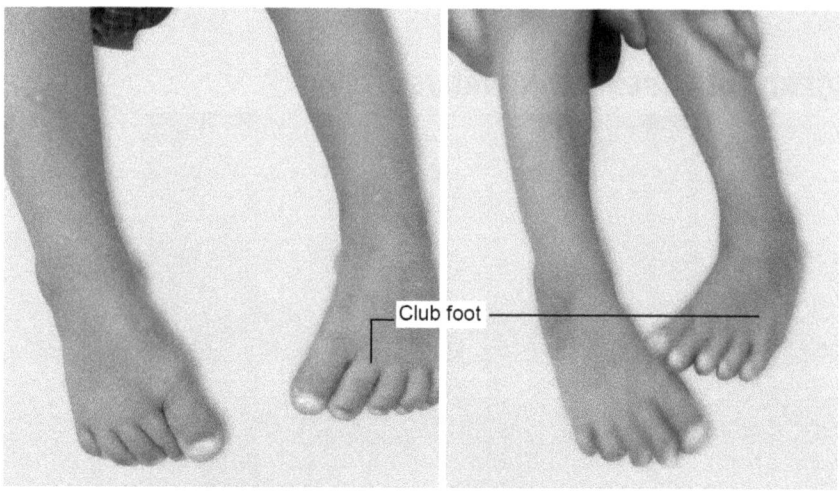
Club foot

Q How do you confirm midfoot varus?
- Varus crease at medial border of foot
- Small, less prominent medial malleoli and large more prominent lateral malleoli
- Small, concave medial border and large convex lateral border

Q How do you confirm forefoot adduction?

By **medial deviation** of all the toes.

Q What investigation do you suggest in CTEV child?

I. X-ray of affected foot (anteroposterior view in planter flexion and lateral in stressed dorsiflexion, also called Kite's view).

Angle measurement:
  a. **Talocalcaneal angle**: Angle formed by the long axis of talus and long axis of calcaneum bone in X-ray plate.
     - In anteroposterior (AP) view: The angle is 35–40°—in normal foot
     - In lateral view: Angle is 30–35°—normal
     - In CTEV: T-C angle is 0° or both axis are parallel to each other.

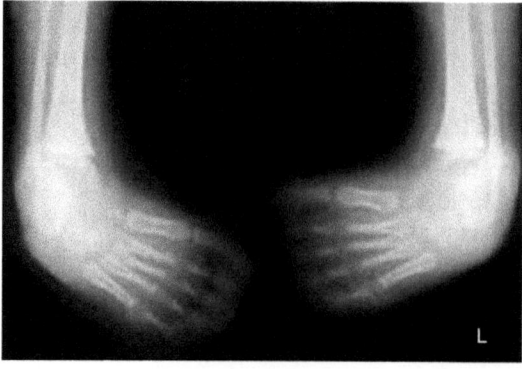

b. **Talo 1st metatarsal angle (TMT):** Angle formed by the long axis of talus and long axis of 1st metatarsal, and measured in AP view only.
   - In normal foot: The angle is 15–20°
   - In **CTEV:** The TMT angle is 5–10°
c. **Lateral view—talotibial angle:** Angle formed by the long axis of talus and long axis of the tibia
   - In normal 70–75° (in CTEV—decrease)
   - In **tibio-calcaneal angle:** Angle formed by the long axis of tibia and long axis of the calcaneum.
   - In normal foot it is 75–85° (in CTEV—angle is decrease)
II. **Podography (foot print in stamp pad):** 1st foot print taken during starting of treatment procedure and in serial interval, as well as after achieving full correction of the deformity (may be after conservative or operative means).
III. **Clinical photography:** Color photographs are taken on serial basis at the beginning and end of treatment procedure.

Q How will you treat a case of CTEV?

Conservative

1. **Manipulation + strapping** (by bandage): Passive manipulation should be started by mother of the child, immediately after birth, as demonstrated by doctor. Manipulation started by mother holding the affected ankle of the child by her left palm and serial correction of equinus by applying reverse force → correction of midfoot varus by valgus force → correction of forefoot by passive abduction force—by the palm of the right hand of mother. At a time 8–10 times serial manipulation done in 3–4 settings per day. After each manipulation cotton bandage should be applied in that corrected position.

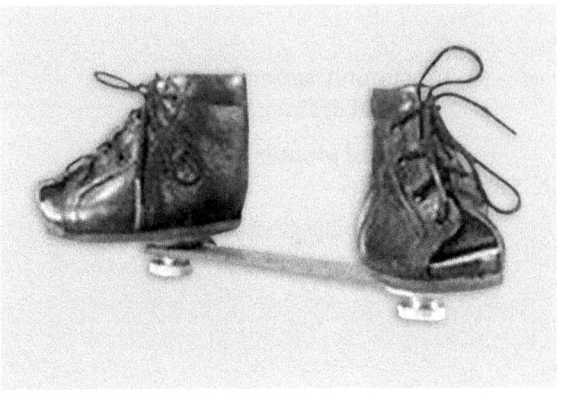

2. **Denis brown splint:** Should be applied after corrective manipulation by mother on daily basis.
3. **Corrective plaster of Paris (POP) cast** above knee at 60° knee flexion should be applied after 1 month of child age. But in Indian scenario, most mothers are not sufficient knowledgeable enough to do manipulation and strapping on regular basis to her child. So most of the cases corrective POP cast is applied on random basis after receiving a child with CTEV, immediately after birth.

⇩

POP cast should be continued for 2 weeks and then cast should be removed to see any skin necrosis, pressure sore and any correction of the deformity—achieved or not. Serial POP casting at 2 weeks interval should be continued till 3 months of age (80% gets corrected by this method).

Surgery: After 3 months if not corrected by conservative method
1. **Tenotomy of tendo-Achilles** tendon at posterior aspect of affected ankle joint, under general anesthesia.
2. **Soft tissue release**—posteromedial soft tissue release (PMSTR)

In PMSTR—inverted hockey stick skin incision given and following structures are usually cut and released.

a. **Capsular release:**
   - Ankle joint (posterior + medial)
   - Talotibial joint
   - Talocalcaneal (whole joint capsule)
   - Talonavicular (superior, inferior, medial) joint

b. **Ligament release:**
   - Spring ligament (talocalcaneonavicular)

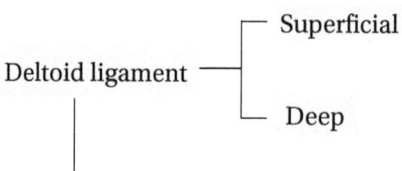

   We cut only **superficial** part of deltoid ligament

   - **Incision at plantar fascia**

c. **Tendon release:**
   - Tendo-Achilles (Z-plasty)

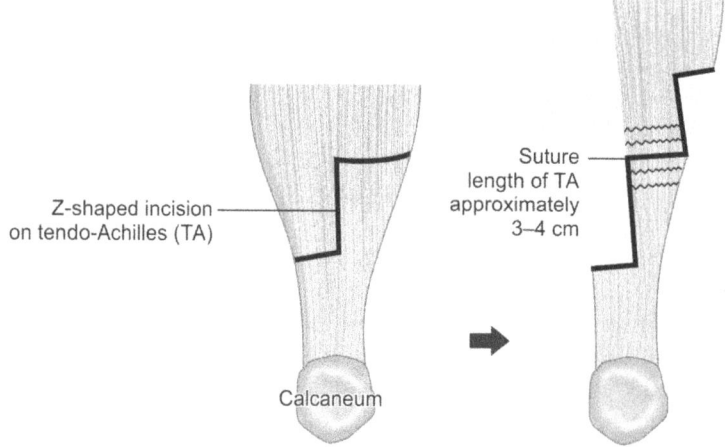

   - Tibialis posterior
   - Flexor hjallucis longus
   - Flexor digitorum longus
   - Master knot of Henry—tight fascio-tendineous structure at the insertion of tibialis posterior at the inferomedial aspect of the base of navicular.

Genetic Disorders

If the deformity is not getting corrected by posteromedial soft tissue release (PMSTR)—extensile release can be done.

Extensile release: PMSTR and release of following structures:
- Lateral capsule of ankle joint + calcaneocubuoid joint capsule
- Fibular collateral ligament.

If deformity more than 2 years (continue till 4 years)
- **Dwyer's osteotomy: Calcaneal wedge osteotomy**—wedge of bone has been removed after preoperative templating of affected calcaneum, after comparing with normal calcaneum
- **Dilwyn Evan's procedure:** Dorsolateral wedge excision of calcaneocuboid joint after preoperative templating.
- **Tarsectomy:** Osteotomy of all the tarsal bones.
- **Metatarsectomy:** Corrective osteotomy of all the metatarsal bones

After 4 years: Extra-articular arthrodesis (**Grice green arthrodesis**)—continue till 10 years.

If deformity more than 10 years—triple arthrodesis: Fusion of the below mention joint after wedge resection.

- Talocalcaneal joint
- Talonavicular joint
- Calcaneocuboid joint

Management of CTEV at any Age

- **JESS fixator:** Joshi's external stabilizing system—multiple K-wire has been passed through the matatarsal, tarsal bone of the affected foot and two thick K-wire has been passed through the upper pole of tibia, along with application of four Joshi's external stabilization system (JESS) distractor rod.

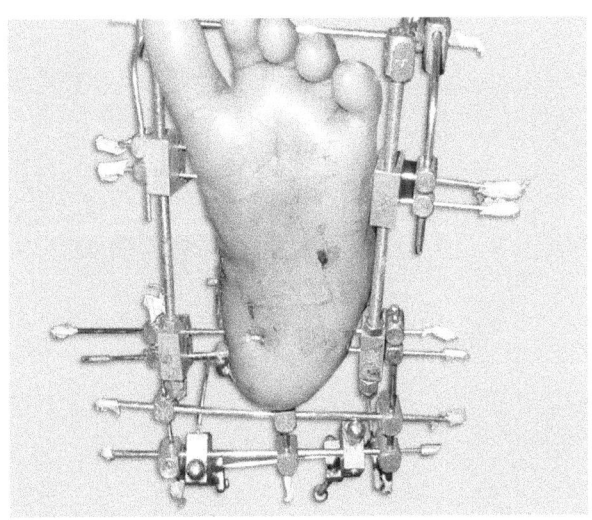

- **Ilizarov's external fixator (ring fixator):** Multiple full ring has been applied in the leg as well as half ring on affected foot along with application of multiple tensioned K-wire and olive wire with different male and female post/bar.

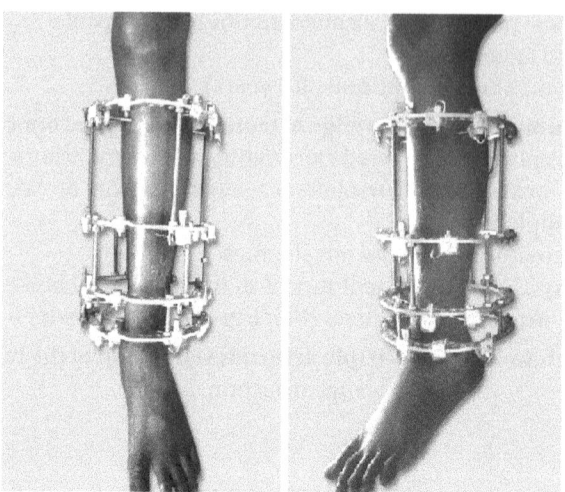

CONGENITAL VERTICAL TALUS

Q How do you diagnose a case of congenital vertical talus?

Talus is vertical in this deformity which is presented by flat foot deformity, since birth.

Investigation: Talocalcaneal angle measurement in X-rays.

Management:
- Corrective foot brace
- Corrective surgery—osteotomy

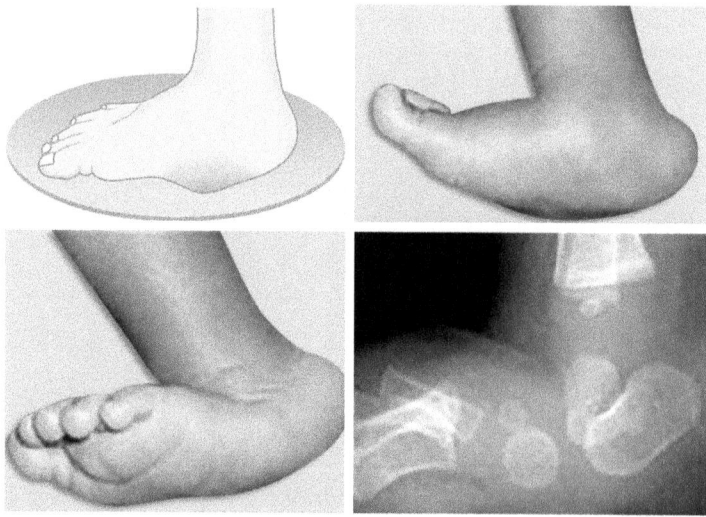

Genetic Disorders

DEVELOPMENTAL DYSPLASIA HIP (DDH)

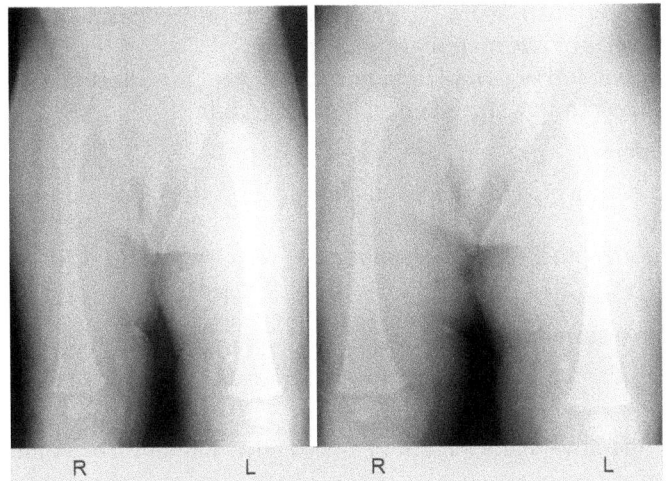

Developmental dysplasia of hip (DDH) at left hip
Old name of DDH is congenital dislocation of hip (CDH)

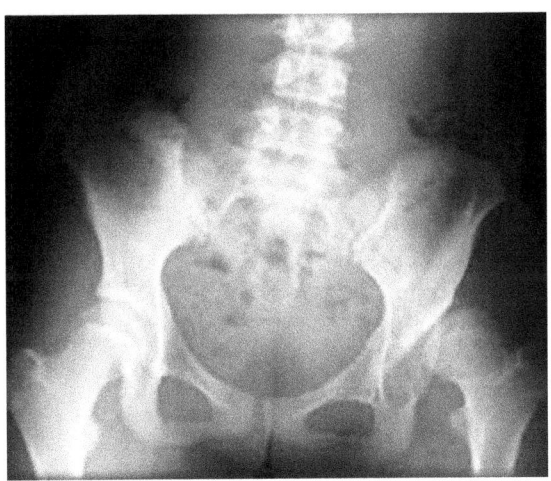

Neglected DDH in an young guy

Q What is the clinical features of DDH?

Clinical features: In child, dislocated femoral head on the posterior aspect of hip joint.
- Immobility of affected
- May be shortening
- Muscle wasting of gluteal and quadriceps muscle
- Deformity of the affected limb (flexion, adduction)
  ⇩
  Confirmed by—Barlow's test and Ortolani's test

Q How will you investigate a case of DDH?

- **Birth history:** Any birth asphyxia or delayed cry of newborn or any pre-eclampsia, associated diabetics or any maternal complication.
- **Clinical features:** Mother complaining of shortness of the affected leg since birth, along with rotational deformity of the affected hip of the child.

Investigation proper:
1. X-ray pelvis with both hip (AP view) and affected hip + thigh (lateral view)
2. MRI of both hip
3. To differentiate any other clinical condition—C-reactive protein (CRP), routine blood test is required.

Q How will you do treatment?

Conservative: Abduction pillow/brace (Milwalcky/Pavlik Harness brace)—up to the age of 6 months of child.

If no correction: Operative management by—corrective derotation osteotomy.

OSTEOGENESIS IMPERFECTA

Q What is the incidence?

- It is one of the most common heritable bone disorders (1 in 20,000).
- It is a connective tissue disorder (defect in collagen type I).

Q What are the most common feature?

- Osteopenia
- Proneness to fracture
- Laxity of ligaments
- Blue sclera
- Crumbling teeth

Q What is the clinical features?

Type I (Mild):
- Majority develop fractures a year or two later
- Deep blue sclera
- General joint laxity

Type II (Severe):
- Lethal—stillborn infant.
- Respiratory difficulties

Type III:
- Diagnosed at birth or more than 6 years
- Kyphoscoliosis
- Triangular face, blue grey sclera
- Wormian bones in skull

Type IV:
- Short stature
- Scoliosis

- Pale blue sclera
- Hearing affected

Q How will you manage a case osteogenesis imperfecta?
- Splinting of fracture
- Open reduction and internal fixation with nail or plate
- Mobilization to prevent osteoporosis
- Multiple osteotomies of deformity correction

SKELETAL DYSPLASIA

Q What are the different types of skeletal dysplasia?
1. Diaphyseal aclasis
2. Achondroplasia
3. Hypochondroplasia
4. Multiple epiphyseal dysplasia
5. Osteopetrosis
6. Proximal focal femoral deficiency

Diaphyseal Aclasis (Hereditary Multiple Exostosis)

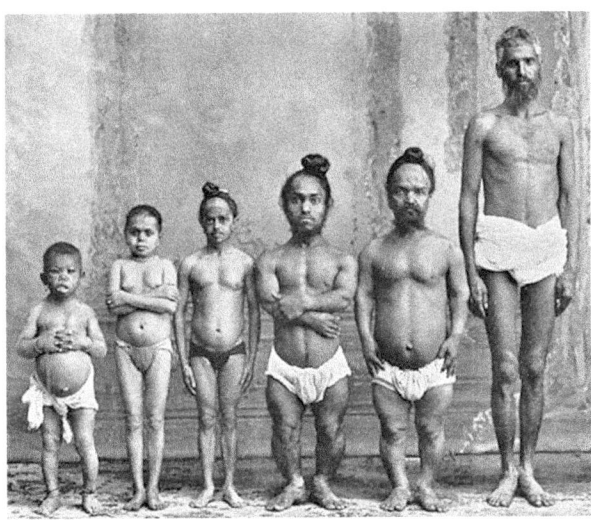

Q What are the clinical features of diaphyseal aclasis?
- Multiple bony lump over long bone, scapula, pelvis.
- Discovering childhood
- Genu varum/valgum or ulnar deviation
- Lump may cause neurogenic symptoms by pressing on nerve.

Q What is the pathology of diaphyseal aclasis?
It is a congenital disorder with autosomal dominant. Basically there are accumulation of multiple solitary exostosis or osteochondroma.

Q **What is the X-ray finding of diaphyseal aclasis?**

Broadening of metaphysis with pedunculated or sessile exostosis.

Q **How do you treat the diaphyseal aclasis?**

- Excision of osteochondromatic mass, when they will put pressure on vessel or nerve.
- Corrective osteotomy for genu varum or valgum.

Achondroplasia (Dwarfism)

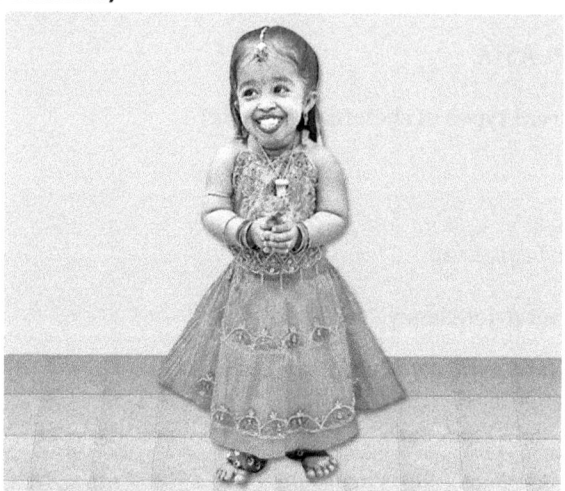

Q **What are the clinical features of achondroplasia?**

It is autosomal dominant disorder.

- Large skull, prominent forehead.
- Shortening of all limbs (mostly proximal segment)
- Too long trunk
- Prominent buttock with flexed hip, knee.
- Bow legs or flexion deformity at elbow.

Q **What is the X-ray finding of achondroplasia?**

Short tubular bone with wide metaphysic and small pelvis.

Q **How do you treat the achondroplasia?**

- Corrective osteotomy for genu varum or valgum.
- Limb lengthening by Ilizarov fixator.
- Excision of mass, when they will put pressure on vessel or nerve.

Hypochondroplasia

Q **Write short notes on hypochondroplasia.**

- It is a autosomal dominant disorder and mild form of achondroplasia.
- Shortness of stature and increased lumbar lordosis is the most common features.
- Other features of achondroplasia may be present.
- Treated by limb lengthening by Ilizarov fixator.

Multiple Epiphyseal Dysplasia

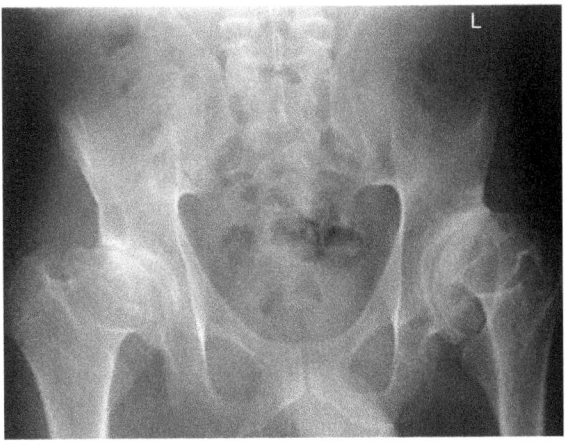

Q Write short note on multiple epiphyseal dysplasia.

Pathology: Autosomal dominant disorder due to abnormal development and ossification of epiphyses.

Clinical features:
- Newborn or child with multiple deformity
- Growth retardation
- Joint pain
- Secondary osteoarthritis
- May be severe crippled

Investigation:
- X-ray—irregular/abnormal epiphyseal line
- Delayed appearance of epiphyses

Treatment by:
- Corrective osteotomy for genu varum or valgum
- Reconstructive surgery for secondary OA.

Osteopetrosis (Marble Bone Disease)

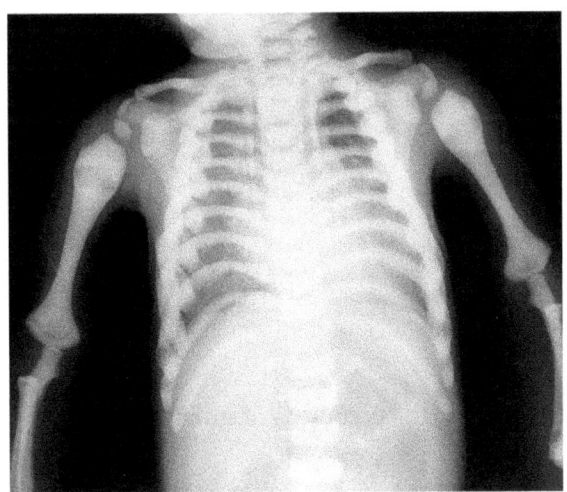

Q Write short notes on osteopetrosis.

Pathology: Autosomal dominant disorder, benign lesion.

Clinical features:
- Patient is asymptomatic usually, diagnosis done after fracture occur.
- Pathological fracture or nerve compression may occur.

X-ray: Increased density of all bones with wide cortex and narrow medullary canal, with sclerosis.

Treatment: Symptomatic

Proximal Focal Femoral Deficiency

Q Write short notes on osteopetrosis.

In this case proximal femur is absent or cartilaginous or shortened.

Clinical features:
- Shortened limb
- Coxa vara

X-ray: Large gap between acetabulum and upper third femur.

Treated by: Limb lengthening by Ilizarov fixator.

CONGENITAL TIBIAL PSEUDOARTHROSIS

Q Write short notes on congenital tibial pseudoarthrosis.
- Anterior bowing of tibia in infant/child usually
- May or not affecting fibula
- X-ray: Gap in shaft of tibia, and looking like fracture non-union.
- Biopsy: Histopathology shows neurofibroma or fibrous dysplasia.
- Treatment by bone grafting/Ilizarov
- Prognosis may not be good, and may lead amputation.

SPINA BIFIDA

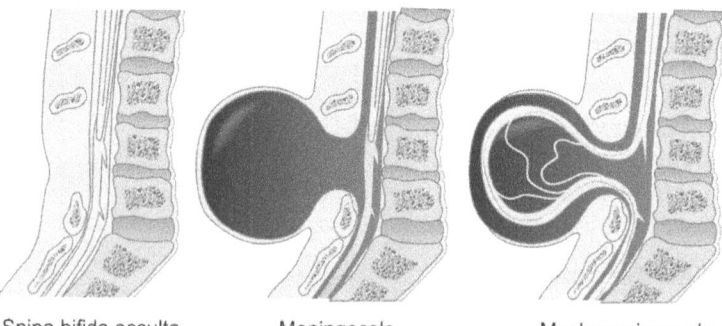

Spina bifida occulta   Meningocele   Myelomeningocele

It is congenital disorder, in which the two halves of the posterior vertebral arch, have failed to fuse.

Q Describe the pathology of spina bifida.

It is of four types:
1. **Spine bifida cystica**
   – Meningocele

- Myelomeninglcele
- Baby presents with paralysis, associated with hip dislocation, talipes, claw toes.

2. **Spine bifida occulta**
   - A midline dimple in overlying skin
   - Tuft of hair
   - Splitting of spinal cord
   - Pigmented nevus (diastometamyelia)
3. **Hydrocephalus**
   - Distal tethering of cord
   - Cause herniation of cerebellum
   - Obstruction in cerebrospinal fluid (CSF) circulation
   - Ventricles and skull enlarges.
4. **Neurological dysfunction**

Q What investigation will you do for spina bifida?
- X-ray whole spine (anteroposterior/lateral view)
- Muscle charting
- MRI brain/spine
- Nerve conduction velocity (NCV) study

Q What treatment will you offer to spina bifida?
- Skin closure—at day 1
- Ventriculocaval shunt—at 1st week
- Stretch and strap—at 1st month
- Orthopedic surgery—according to need
- Urogenital surgery—if needed.

CHAPTER 2

Infection

OSTEOMYELITIS

Q What do you mean by osteomyelitis?
- Osteo—bone
- Myel—muscle
- Itis—inflammation/infection

Q What are the types?
There are two types of osteomyelitis:
1. Acute
2. Chronic

Acute Osteomyelitis

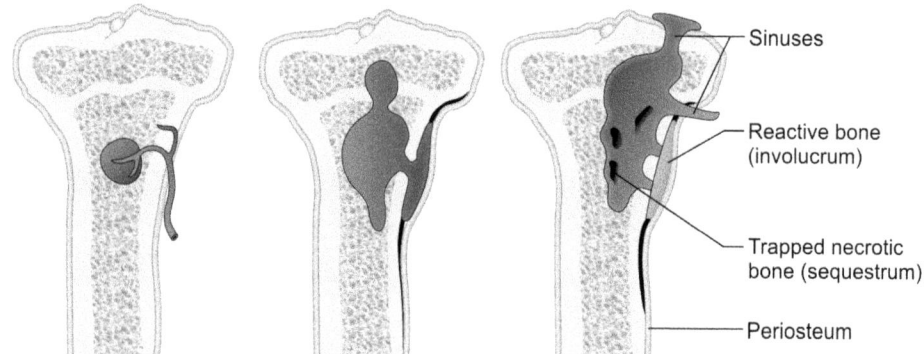

Q What are the clinical features?

Symptoms:
- Usually in child
- High fever
- Pain, swelling of affected limb
- Inability to move or walk

Signs:
- Local tenderness +++ of the affected
- Swelling +++ of the affected area of the limb with redness with tense
- Range of movements of nearby joint—restricted

- Lymphadenopathy ++
- Features of toxemia may be present

In adults: Common site—dorsal spine and/or hip.

Q Describe the pathology of acute osteomyelitis.

- Inflammation
- Suppuration
- Necrosis
- Reactive new bone formation
- Resolution and healing
- Most common organism—*Staphylococcus aureus*

Child <4 years: *Haemophilus influenzae*

Patient of sickle cell disease: *Salmonella*

Most common route: Hemotogenous.

Q How will you investigate the case acute osteomyelitis?

- From history of fever, pain at limb with restriction of movement of the affected limb.
- Plain X-ray: No abnormality of bone in 1st to 2nd week except soft tissue swelling.
  - After 2nd week: Periosteal new bone may be seen with classic sign of pyogenic osteomyelitis.
  - Late: Regional osteoporosis with increase bone density.
- MRI: Differentiate between pus and blood
- Blood:

Hemoglobin (HB%)—↓

Total leukocyte count (TLC)— ↑↑

Erythrocyte sedimentation rate (ESR)—↑

C-reactive protein (CRP)—raised

Q What could be the differential diagnosis?

- Cellulitis
- Acute rheumatism
- Sickle cell crisis
- Gaucher's disease

Treatment:

- Treatment for pain by nonstroidal anti-inflammatory drugs (NSAIDs) and maintain of hydration by normal saline [intravenous fluid (IVF)]
- Splintage by skin traction or by Thomas
- Intravenous antibiotics immediately

If no response:

- Surgery: Incision given on the most tense area of the swelling
- Dissection done layer after layer
- Making cortical window at the diaphysis of the affected bone
- Drainage of pus from

- Debridement done thoroughly and wash with normal saline
- Wound closed keeping a drain inside bony cavity
- Splintage of the affected limb with advised to bed rest
- And culture sensitivity of the aspirated pus and choice of antibiotic IV accordingly for 3 weeks.

Chronic Osteomylitis

It is sequel of acute osteomyelitis, but nowadays, frequently follows open fracture and surgery.

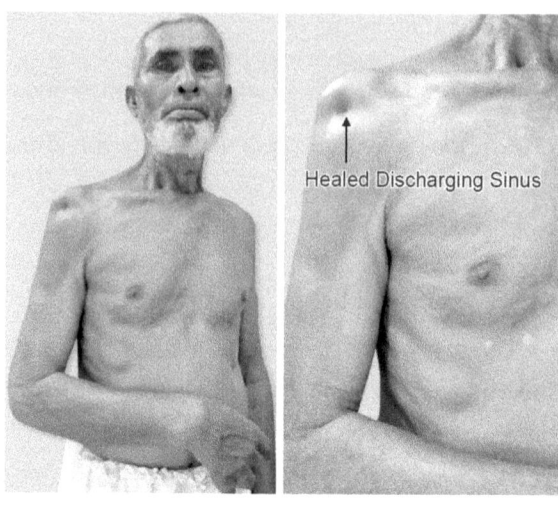
Healed Discharging Sinus

Q Describe the pathology of chronic osteomyelitis.

Common organisms:
- *Staphylococcus aureus*
- *E. coli*
- *Pseudomonas*

At the infection site, bone is destroyed (osteolysis)
↓
Formation of cavity with pus and dead bone (**sequestrum**) and surrounded by vascularized healthy bone (**involucrum**)
↓
Beyond that area osteosclerosis with a discharging sinus at skin.

Q What is the clinical features of chronic osteomyelitis?

Symptoms:
- History of open fracture or surgery
- Pain, mild fever, discharging sinus

Signs: Local tenderness, discharging sinus—skin is puckered, inverted fixed to the underlying bone with color of discharged according to causative bacteria.
- Range of movement of nearby joint—restricted
- Muscle wasting of affected limb +
- Affected bone—thickened, broadened, irregular surface
- Shortening of limb ±

Q How will you investigate chronic osteomyelitis?
- **Blood:** HB%, WBC, ESR
- **X-ray:** Bone resorption markedly osteolysis with osteosclerosis.
    - Area of osteoporosis
    - Periosteal thickening/reactions
        - Sunray specules

- Onion peel appearance
- Codmann's triangle
- **CT/MRI:** For operative planning and to see the extent of bone destruction
- **Treatment:**
  - Pus for culture sensitivity
  - And IV antibiotic accordingly for long term (6 months)
  - ASD locally

If no response: Operation

Q What surgery will you do?

- Excision of sinus tract
- Sequestrectomy—removal of dead bone
- Saucerization—make a saucer like bony cavity after thorough curettage of the bony cavity, along with removal of pus, debrima and unhealthy infected granulation tissue.
- Debridement of bony cavity
- Wash with hydrogen peroxide and normal saline and antibiotic solution.
- Cavity filled with antibiotic impregnated bone graft.
- Stay sutures given on skin after keeping a drain inside the cavity.

SEPTIC ARTHRITIS OF HIP

Q Describe the pathology of septic arthritis.

Common presentation in children pathology → Septic foci → Lodge at major joints
Hematogenous route
Staphylococcus aureus in adults
Haemophilus in neonates
Streptococcus in neonates

What are the clinical features?

- High fever, loss of movement of the affected limb and child may be in toxemia.
- On examination—local tenderness around hip joint.
- Restriction of movement in any direction is painful.

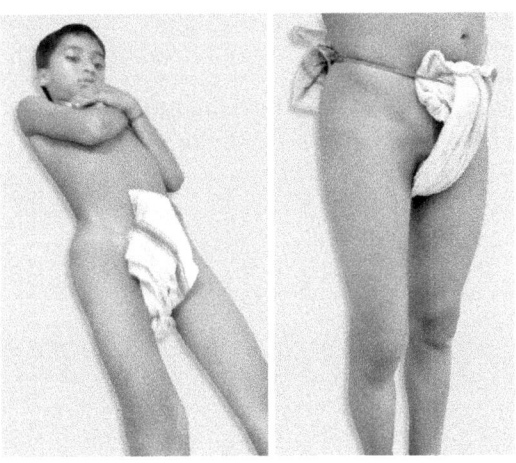

Q How will you investigate septic arthritis?
- X-ray—no change, if it is early (after 3 weeks)
- USG of the affected
- MRI of the affected joint—collection of fluid and/or pus

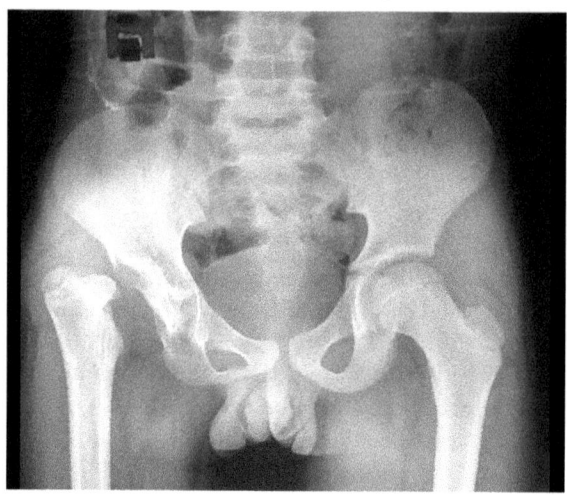

Q How will you treat septic arthritis of hip?
- After clinical assessment of hip and general condition of child.
- Routine blood picture and emergency ultrasonography (USG) of affected.
- Drainage of pus in a sterile condition° or aseptic aspiration° Frank pus come out° followed by exploration.

ARTHROTOMY

By anterior approach of hip joint—Smith-Peterson approach to hip
- Dissection done layer after
- Hip joint capsule
- Joint capsule cut anteriorly
- Remove all pus, debrima
- Culture sensitivity of pus
- Tissue biopsy (*H. pylori* examination) of hip joint capsule
- IV antibiotics, rest, immobilization by skin traction for 2–3 weeks.

CHAPTER 3

Rheumatic Disorders

RHEUMATOID ARTHRITIS

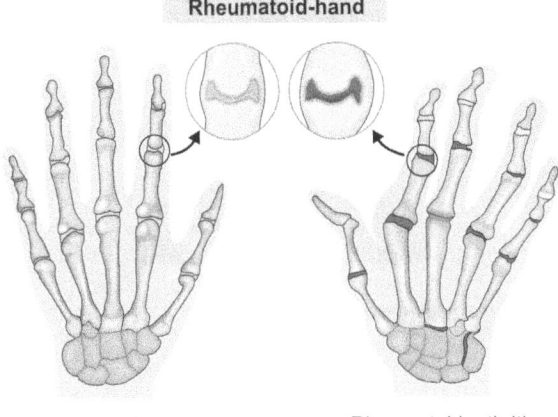

It is the most common cause of chronic inflammatory joint diseases.

Q What is pathology of rheumatoid arthritis?

Intra-articular:
- Stage of synovitis
- Destructive stage—erosion of articular cartilage osteoclastic resorption.
- Stage of deformity—auto-rupture of capsule/tendons.

Extra-articular:
- Rheumatoid nodule
- Lymphadenopathy
- Splenomegaly
- Myopathy/neuropathy

Q What are the clinical features of rheumatoid arthritis?

Symptoms:
- Women of 30–40 years, are commonly affected.
- Pain, swelling, deformity of hand, knee and elbow with morning stiffness.

Signs (complaining of):
- Polyarthralgia
- Small joints of hands are swollen, tender

- Deformity of hand/foot—metatarsophalangeal (MTP) or interphalangeal (IP) joints may be dislocated.

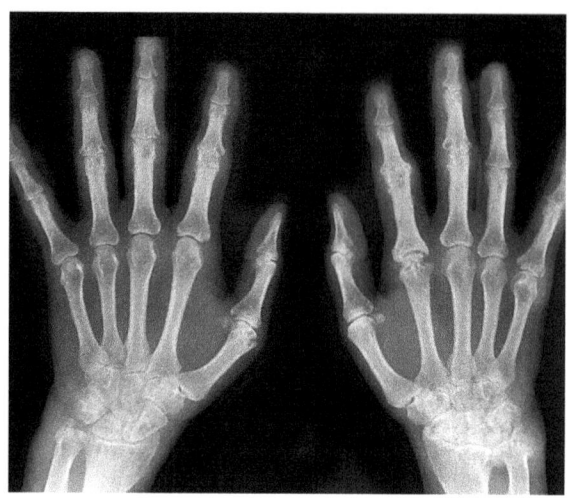

Q How will you investigate rheumatoid arthritis?

Blood:
- Hb%—decreased
- ESR—raised
- RA factor: +ve (seropositive—80% case)
- Antistreptolysin O (ASO) titer: +ve
- ANF: +/−

X-ray of hands—showing periarticular osteopenia/osteoporosis

Synovial biopsy—for *H. pylori* examination

Treatment:
- Rest
- Nonsteroidal anti-inflammatory drugs (NSAIDs)
- Disease-modifying antirheumatic drugs (DMARDs):
  - Methotrexate
  - Sulfasalazine
  - Salazopyrin
  - Hydroxychloroquine
  - Leflunamide
- Systemic corticosteroids
- Corticosteroids intrasynovial injection

If no response: Correction of deformity by osteotomy or replacement arthroplasty (total hip replacement/total knee replacement/total elbow replacement).

ANKYLOSING SPONDYLITIS

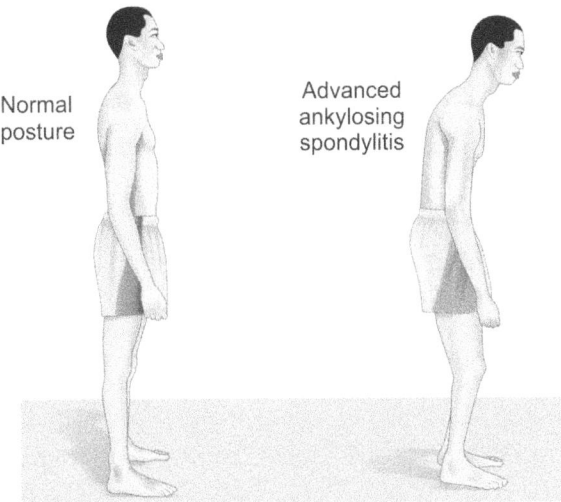

Normal posture

Advanced ankylosing spondylitis

Generalized chronic inflammatory diseases, mainly affecting spine and sacroiliac joints, commonly occur in young male.

Q What is the diagnostic criteria?
- History of low backache
- Limitations of range of movement of lumbar spine and cervical spine.
- Limited chest expansion
- Radiograph—sacroiliitis and bamboo spine
- Blood: HLA B-27 is positive.

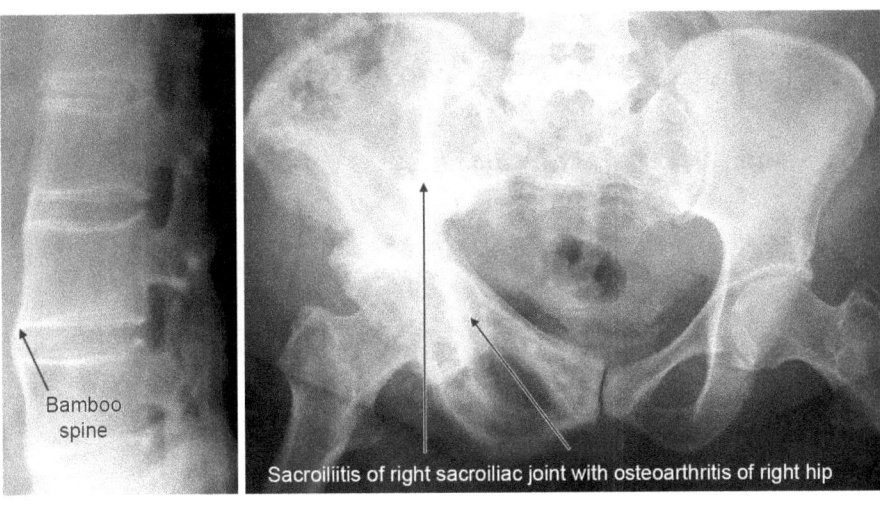

Bamboo spine

Sacroiliitis of right sacroiliac joint with osteoarthritis of right hip

Q How will you treat ankylosing spondylitis?
- Spinal extension exercise
- NSAIDs (indomethacin)
- Surgery: According to stiffness of joint
  - Stiffness of hip—total hip
  - Stiffness of spine—cervical/lumbar osteotomy.

OTHER RHEUMATIC DISORDERS
- Reiter's syndrome (urethritis, arthritis, conjunctivitis)
- Psoriatic arthritis (polyarthralgia, i.e., psoriasis)
- Juvenile chronic arthritis
- Enteropathic arthritis (with Crohn's disease or ulcerative colitis).

CHAPTER 4
Crystal Deposition Disorder

GOUT

Disorder of purine metabolism, characterized by hyperuricemia and recurrent synovitis.

Q Describe the pathology of gout.

Deposition of urate crystals in connective tissue and articular cartilage.

Common sites: Metatarsophalangeal joint of great toe, tendo-Achillis, olecranon bursae, ear pinna.

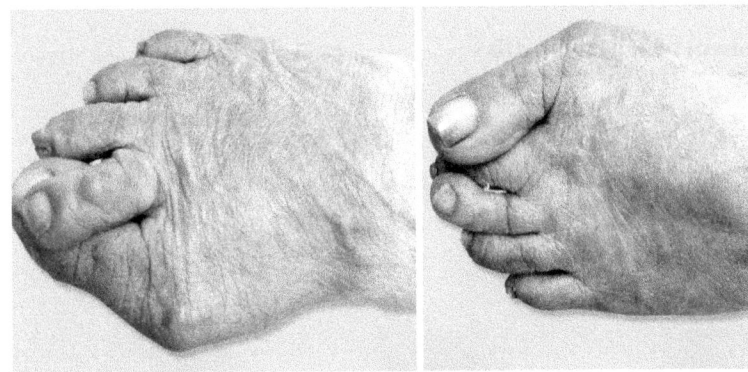

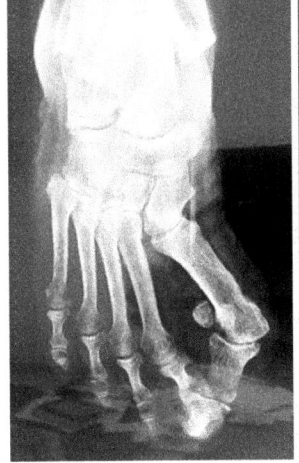
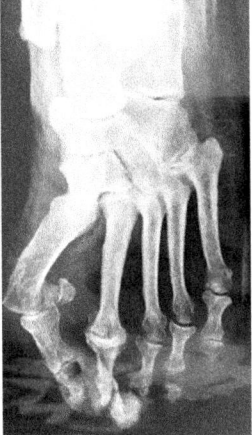

Gouty tophi at metatarsophalangeal joint.

Crystal Deposition Disorder

Q Describe clinical features of gout.
- Usually male—40 years
- Joint pain suddenly
- Swelling local tenderness at
- Skin is red and shiny
- Later—tophi, renal calculi, etc.

Q How will you investigate gouty arthritis?
- X-ray: Narrowing of joint space and secondary osteoarthritis (OA)
- Blood for uric acid: Increased +/- (not diagnostic)
- Synovial fluid analysis: Negatively birefringent urate crystals in fluid.

Q What is differential diagnosis of gouty arthritis?
- Cellulitis
- Reiter's disease
- Pseudo-gout (pyrophosphate crystal deposition) common in women and large joint affection
- Rheumatoid arthritis

Q What is the treatment of gouty arthritis?
- Rest
- NSAIDs
- Colchicine—less effective
- Allopurinol—in chronic gout (drug of choice)
- Feburic acid—the latest drug (**Febuxostat**).

CHAPTER 5: Osteoarthritis

Q Define osteoarthritis.

Chronic joint disorder, characterized by destruction of articular cartilage with new growth of bone and cartilage.

Types:
1. Primary (idiopathic)
2. Secondary (commonest to surgery/fracture/disease)

Q Describe pathology of osteoarthritis.

Progressive cartilage destruction leads to:
- Subarticular cyst formation
- Sclerosis of joint
- Osteophyte formation
- Capsular fibrosis

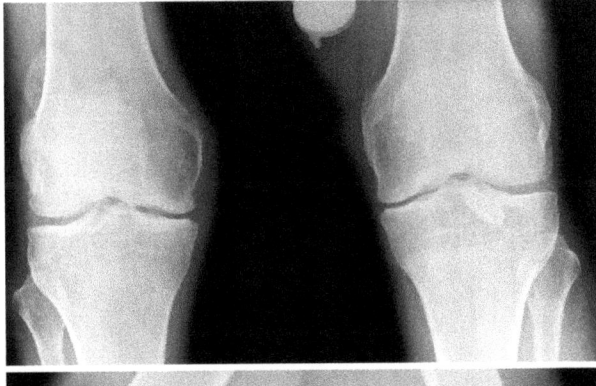

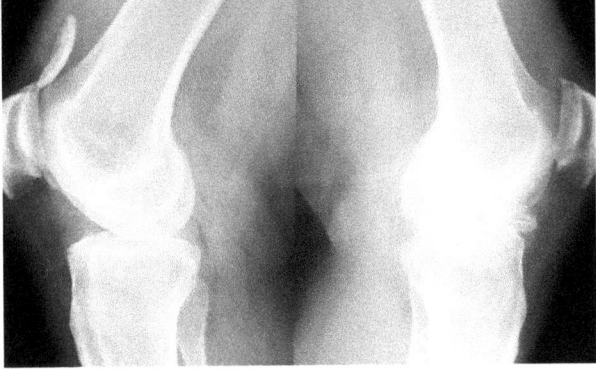

Q What are the clinical features of osteoarthritis?
- Usually middle age
- Pain, swelling of affected joint
- Stiffness of joint
- Deformity (OA knee)—genu varum and genu valgum
- Loss of function (difficult walking/strain, climbing)
- Muscle wasting
- Late—sensorial thickening

GENU VARUM

Intercondylar distance (normal 6–8 cm)—increased and bowing of both the knees and legs but intermalleolar distance (normal 4–6 cm)—decreased.

GENU VALGUM OR KNOCK KNEE (REVERSE OF GENU VARUM)

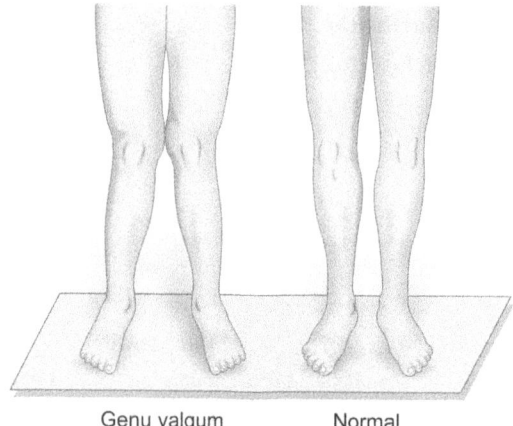

Genu valgum   Normal

In this deformity both the knee are touching each other and intermalleolar distance are increased.

Q What are the investigations and treatment in genu valgum?
Investigation:
- X-ray: Joint narrowing, osteophytes, sclerosis
- CT/MRI: Cartilage destruction

Treatment:

Early:
- NSAIDs
- Mobilizing exercise
- Weight loss
- Dietary supplement: Glucosamine, chondroitin, diacerin

Late:
- Realignment osteotomy or

- Arthroplasty in old age
  - Total hip replacement (THR)
  - Total knee replacement (TKR)

TOTAL KNEE REPLACEMENT

After clinical and radiological assessment of the patients.
- Strict asepsis
- Anterior midline
- Medial parapatellar incision given
- Removal of osteophytes, damage cartilages, Torn ligaments
- Soft tissue balancing
- Tibial cut followed by femoral cut done
- Resurfacing of patella
- Component trail
- PCL sacrificing tibial and femoral prosthesis put along with bone cement
- Range of movement of knee checked.

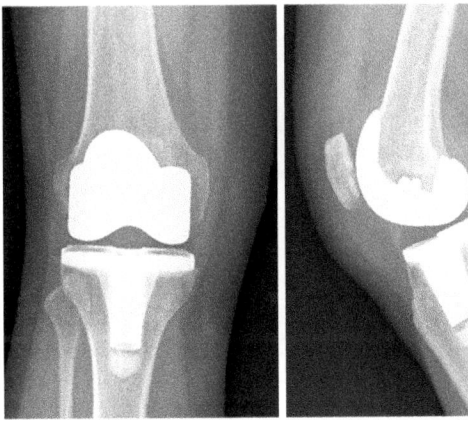

- Wound close layer after layer, after putting drain
- Pressure bandage (RJ Last) applied
- Q excise started from day of surgery, when patient got pain relief
- Standing and walking started from 2nd postoperative day, according to tolerance of patient.

CHAPTER 6

Avascular Necrosis (Osteonecrosis)

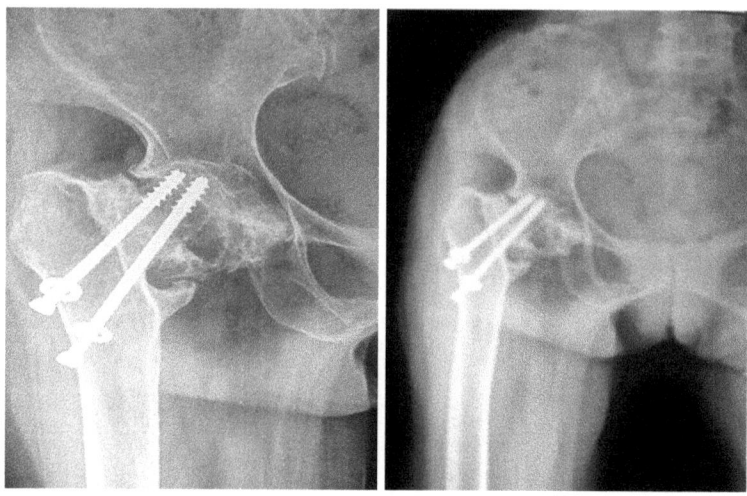

Avascular necrosis (AVN) of femoral head after fracture neck of femur with fixation (by CHS)

Q Describe the causes of avascular necrosis.

The causes are two types:
1. Primary—idiopathic
2. Secondary—to fracture:
   - Dislocation
   - Infection
   - Vasculitis
   - Sickle cell disease
   - Alcohol abuse and corticosteroid prolonged intake

Q Describe pathogenesis, clinical features and investigation of AVN.

Pathogenesis:
- Arterial insufficiency—venous occlusion
- Intraosseous capillary occlusion—intravascular capillary occlusion

Clinical features:
- Pain, stiffness of joint
- Local tenderness
- Fixed deformity
- Gross restriction of movement of joint.

Investigation:
- X-ray:
  - Increased bone density (sclerosis)
  - Crescent sign (+ve) 60% case
  - Collapse of a bone segment
- MRI: Signal intensity—early detection (in stage I)

Q Describe the classification of AVN.

Classification of AVN by Ficat and Arlet (1980):
Stage 1: Preclinical phase of ischemia (detected by MRI).

Stage 2: Painful and characterized by radiograph.

Stage 3: Clear radiological changes of AVN

Stage 4: Collapse of articular cartilage and secondary osteoarthritis (OA)

Q How will you treat AVN?

Stage I and II: Operative
- Medullary decompression
- Bone grafting in femoral neck

Stage III and IV:
- Osteotomy (for realignment)
- Arthroplasty (total hip replacement, total knee replacement)
- Arthrodesis (mostly for ankle)

TOTAL HIP REPLACEMENT
- After clinical and radiological assessment of the strict asepsis
- Anterior lateral approach (modified Watson–Jones approach)
- Dissection done between tensor fasciae latae and gluteus medius
- Hip joint capsule cut at inverted T-shaped manner
- Removal of osteophytes, damage cartilages, Torn ligaments
- Soft tissue balancing
- Femoral cut followed by acetabular reaming done
- Component trail given
- Acetabular and femoral prosthesis put along with bone cement
- Range of movement of hip checked after relocation.
- Wound close layer after layer, after putting drain
- Pressure bandage applied
- Hip and knee exercise started from day of surgery, when patient got pain relief.
- Standing and walking started from 2nd postoperative day, according to tolerance of patient.

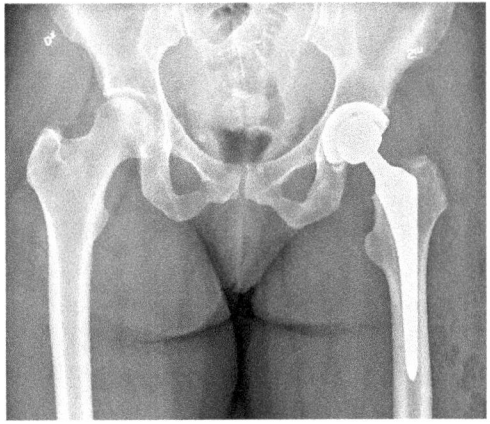

CHAPTER 7
Metabolic and Endocrine Disorders

OSTEOPOROSIS

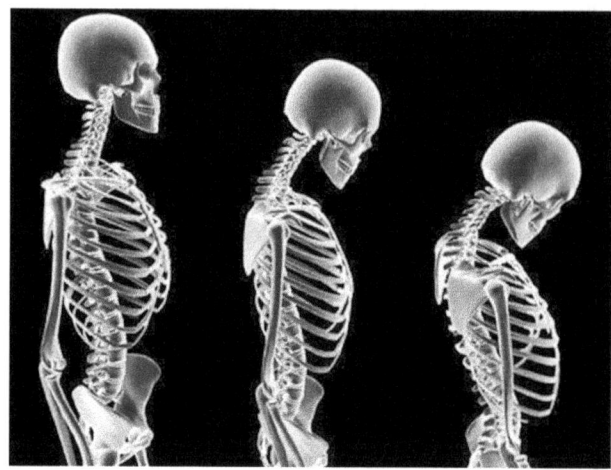

Q Describe type, clinical features, and preventive measures of osteoporosis.

There are two types:
1. Primary (postmenopausal)
2. Secondary (prolonged immobilization, debilitating disease, multiple myeloma, alcohol)

Clinical features:
- Commonly in female (>45 years)
- Complaining of low backache
- Increased kyphosis at dorsal spine
- May be fracture distal radius after minor injury.

Prevention:
- Intake of calcium-rich diet (1,500 mg/day calcium)
- High level of physical activities
- Avoid smoking/alcohol
- Estrogen replacement therapy after hysterectomy

Q How will you investigate and treat osteoporosis?

Investigation:
- Blood:
  - Vitamin D_3 level—decreased
  - Hb%—decreased

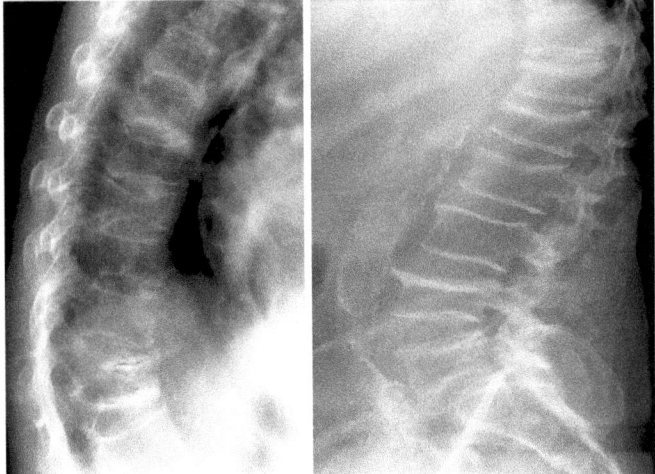

- X-ray: Loss of trabecular marking in femoral neck and vertebral bodies.
- MRI of spine: Compression of vertebral body.

Treatment:
- Rest and dietary calcium supplement
- Gradual mobilizing exercise
- Vitamin D_3 supplementation
- Calcitonin nasal spray or injection
- Bisphosphonates
  - Alendronate
  - Risedronate
  - Ibandronate

If fracture: Stabilization of fracture fragment by appropriate implant
- Dynamic hip screw (DHS)
- Dynamic condylar screw (DCS)
- Cannulated hip screw (CHS)
- Interlocking nail
- Titanium elastic nail screw (TENS)
- Broad or narrow dynamic compression plate (DCP)

RICKETS

Due to inadequate mineralization of bone in children.

Describe etiology of rickets.
- Calcium deficiency in diet
- Hypophosphatemia
- Vitamin D metabolism defects (nutritional, decrease sunlight exposure)
- Intestinal malabsorption syndrome
- Liver disease
- Anticonvulsant drug

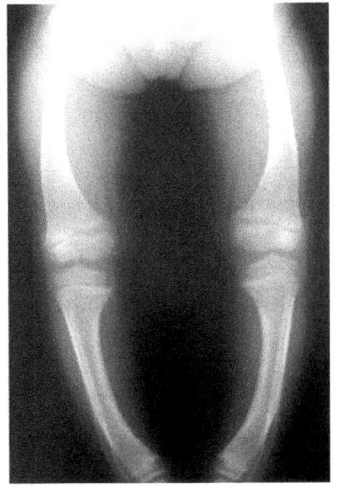

Q What are the clinical feature of rickets?
- Thickening of epiphysis of knee, ankle and wrist.
- Tibial bowing, coxa vara or bending/fractures of long bones
- Rickety rosary—enlargement of costochondral junction
- Craniotabes—frontal bossing, depressed alar nasae
- Pigeon-shaped chest
- Harrisson's sulcus (lateral indentation) in chest
- Protuberant abdomen
- Spinal deformity

Q How will you investigate rickets?
- **X-ray:**
    - Thickening, widening of growth plate
    - Cupping metaphysic
    - Bowing of diaphysis
- **Blood biochemistry:**
    - Calcium level—decrease
    - Phosphate level—decrease
    - Alkaline phosphate level—decease
    - 25(OH)-cholecalciferol—decrease, in vitamin D deficiency
- **Biopsy:** Osteoid seams are wider and extensive.

Q What treatment will you give in rickets?
- **Conservative:**
    - Vitamin D and calcium enriched diet
    - Exposure to sunlight
    - Oral supplementation of calcium and vitamin D_3 (1,000 IU/day)
    - Injection arachitol (6 lac IU/week) for 6 weeks at least
- **Operative:**
    - Corrective valgus/varus osteotomy according to deformity
    - Open reduction internal fixation (ORIF) with titanium elastic nail system (TENS)/nail or
    - Limited contact dynamic compression plate (DCP) [limited contact dynamic compression plate (LCDCP)], if pathological fracture occur.

Vitamin D Deficient Rickets

Q Write short notes of vitamin D deficient rickets.
Etiology: Due to dietary deficiency in vegetarian and old people and decrease sunlight exposure.

Clinical features: Like rickets

Treatment: By vitamin D_3 (1,000 IU)/per day and calcium supplement in intestinal malabsorption.

Hypophosphatemic Rickets

Q Write short notes on hypophosphatemic rickets

Here serum calcium is normal but mineralization is defective.

In familial hypophosphatemic rickets (vitamin D resistant):
- Most common form of rickets
- X-linked genetic disorder
- Dwarfism child (M > F)
- X-ray—shows marked epiphyseal changes
- No secondary hyperparathyroidism
- Treatment by large dose of vitamin D_3 (60,000 IU/day + up to 4 g of inorganic phosphate/day) and corrective osteotomy in deformity.

In adult hypophosphatemic rickets:
- Polyarthralgia with unexplained bone loss.
- Treatment by phosphate, calcium and vitamin D_3.

Hyperparathyroidism

Q Write short notes on hyperparathyroidism.

These are of two types:
1. Primary
2. Secondary

Clinical features:
- Patients are 40–65 years women (F:M = 2:1)
- Initially asymptomatic, but later develops anorexia, nausea, pain abdomen, muscle weakness, depression
- May develop polyuria
- Polyarthralgia due to chondrocalcinosis
- Osteoporosis
- Bone cyst—leads to pathological fracture

Investigation:
- X-ray shows subperiosteal bone resorption, in middle phalanges, clavicle, and proximal humerus.
- Blood—hypercalcemia, hypophosphatemia, increased parathyroid hormone (PTH) and alkaline phosphatase.

Treatment:
- Adequate
- Decrease calcium intake
- If any renal pathology like calculi, nephrocalcinosis—removal of calculi, nephrectomy
- Parathyroidectomy—if persistent renal symptoms and severe osteoporosis.

Renal Rickets

Q Write short notes on renal rickets.

- Patient with chronic renal failure leads to diffuse bone changes causing phosphate and aluminum retention and causing uremia.
- Clinical features:
  - Osteoporosis
  - Osteosclerosis
  - Osteomalacia
  - Features of hyperparathyroidism
  - In child—presented with pasty faced, stunted growth, myopathy, and rachitic deformity.
- Treatment with large dose of vitamin D_3 (5,00,000 IU at least) and epiphysiolysis.

CHAPTER 8

Bone Tumors

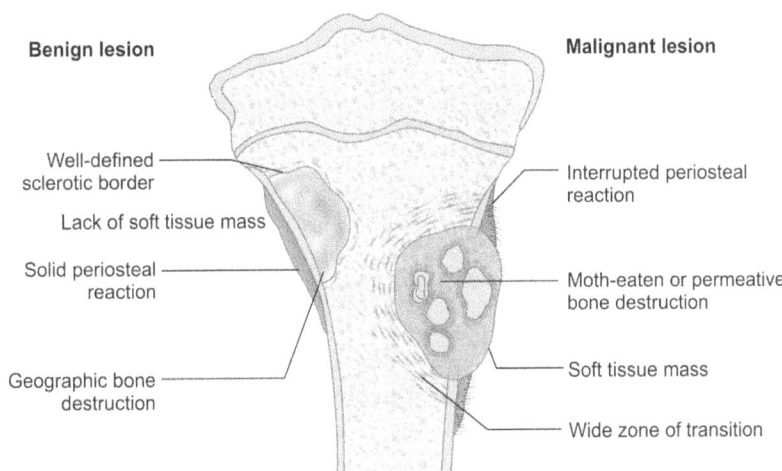

Q Enumerate benign and malignant bone tumors.

Benign:
- Osteoid osteoma
- Fibroma
- Osteochondroma (exostosis)
- Giant cell tumor
- Eosinophilic granuloma and hemangioma

Malignant:
- Osteosarcoma
- Chondrosarcoma
- Ewing's sarcoma
- Multiple myeloma
- Malignant giant cell tumor (GCT)

OSTEOCHONDROMA OR EXOSTOSIS

Q Describe clinical features, investigation, pathology, investigation and treatment of osteochondroma.
- Benign tumor arising from diaphysis long bone of a nearby joint.
- Most common site—long bone of knee, wrist, elbow, ankle.

Clinical features:
- Teenage/young adult
- No pain
- Only swelling (insidious onset)
- May result deformity
- Palpation of mass:
  - Cauliflower-like swelling
  - Round or oval solid mass
  - Grow away form joint

Investigation:

Plain X-ray:
- Pedunculated bony mass arising from cortex of a diaphysis.
- Metaphyseal junction with calcification of cartilage cap.

Pathology:
- History and physical examination—cap of hyaline cartilage over the bony mass.
- MRI—to rule out neurovascular compression by mass.

Treatment:
- Observation—if small
- If growing—excision of the mass along with stalk.

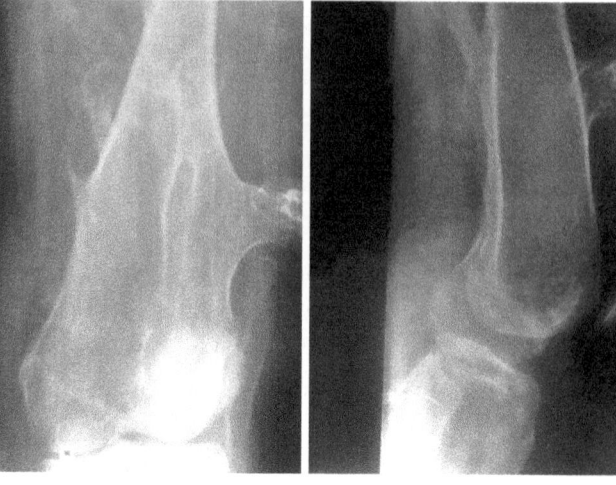

SIMPLE BONE CYST

Q Write short note of simple bone cyst.

Benign mass occur during childhood form metaphysis of long bone.

Common site: Proximal humerus, distal femur.

Pathology: Straw color yellow fluid, fibrous capsule +/− giant cell.

Clinical features:
- Swelling, no pain, no local tenderness
- Pathological fracture may happen.

Treatment:
- Usually heal spontaneously
- If increases size gradually—then curettage and bone graft

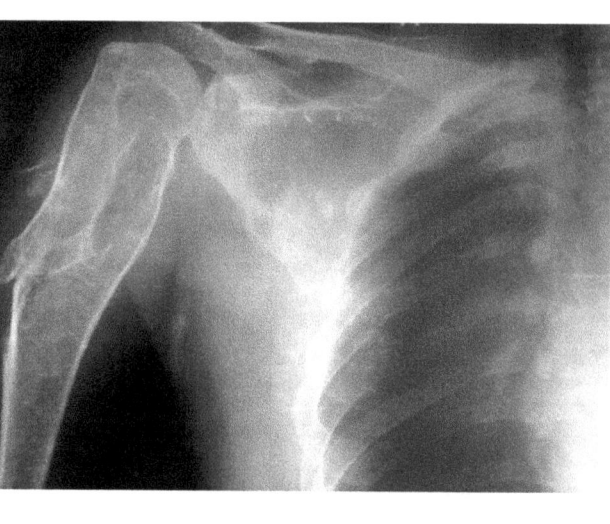

Bone Tumors

ANEURYSMAL BONE CYST

Q Write short note on aneurysmal bone cyst.

These occur in middle age group from metaphysis.

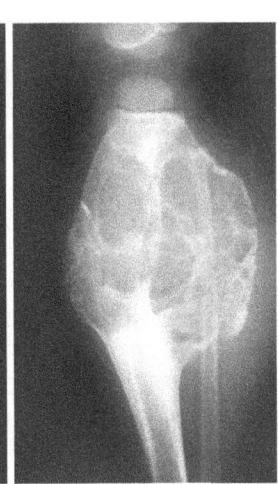

Clinical features:
- Pain, swelling, around a joint
- Common sites of swelling:
  - Proximal tibia, humerus, femur
  - Distal femur and tibia
- Local tenderness +ve

Investigation:
- *X-ray:*
  - Well-defined radiolucent cyst
  - Trabeculated cyst
- *CT/MRI:* To detect cortical break.

Pathology: Contains blood with a fibrous capsule +/- giant cell

Treatment: Curettage + bone graft or bone cement

EOSINOPHILIC GRANULOMA

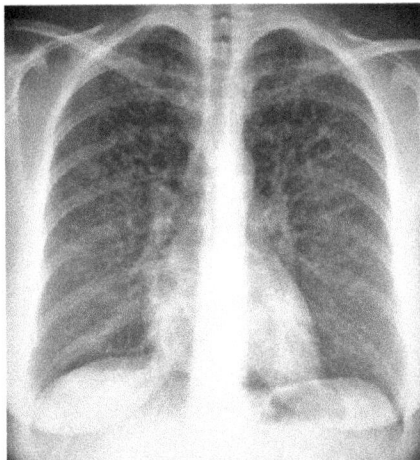
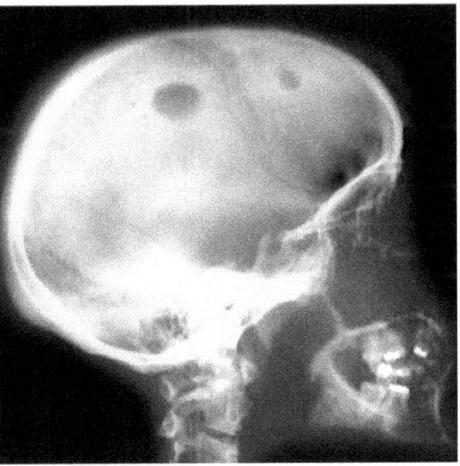

Q Write short notes on eosinophilic granuloma.

Clinical features:
- Cystic lesions in flat bone or metaphysis of long bone, usually in child.
- Complaining of—pain, swelling
- Pathological fracture may occur

Investigation:
- *X-ray:* Well demarcated, radiculated area with bone metaphysis with sclerosis, occurring skull vertebrae also.
- *MRI:* To differentiate spinal cord compression.

Treatment:
- Usually heal spontaneously
- Operation
  - To obtain biopsy
  - If lesion increased in size—complete excision.

GIANT CELL TUMOR

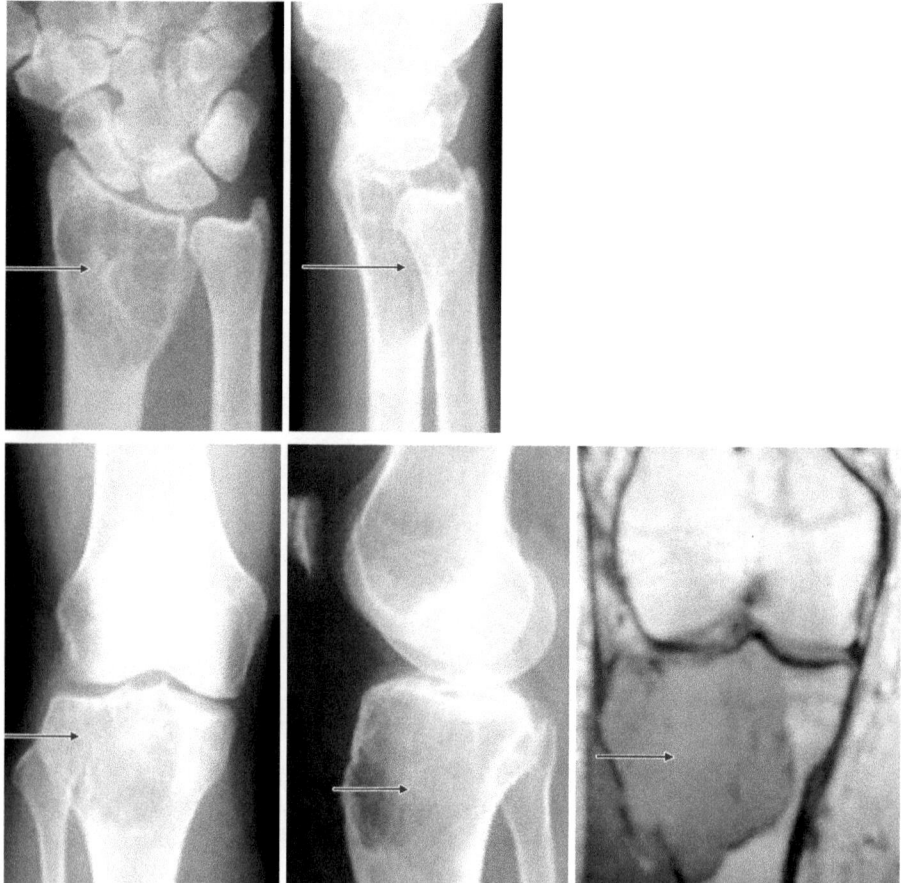

Q Write short note on giant cell tumor (GCT).

Clinical features:
- History: 3rd to 4th decade, usually female (2:1)
- Pain and swelling mostly knee, ankle, elbow, shoulder (mild to moderate) and severe restriction of movement.

Sign:
- Swelling away from joint around joint of a long bone.
- Tenderness positive—egg cell crackling sound.

Investigation:
- Radiology—X-ray and MRI—soap bubble appearance
- Bony mass with enlarged cortex, i.e., seepage test +ve
- Confirm by MRI—due to any breakage or soft tissue involvement or any neurovascular involvement, area of osteolysis and sclerosis
- Confirm by bone biopsy—wide bore needle biopsy
- Incisional biopsy confirm—at the junction of malignant bone and healthy tissue—should be done by an expert.

Histopatholgy: Multi nucleated osteoclast type giant cells, sheets of uniform oval mononuclear cells.

Treatment: Curettage and bone cement to fill the tumor cavity.

MALIGNANT TUMOR OF BONE

Enumerate malignant bone tumor with their occurrence age.
- Osteosarcoma (2nd decade)
- Ewing sarcoma (1st decade)
- Chondrosarcoma (4th–5th decade)
- Multiple Myeloma (6th–7th decade)
- Malignant giant cell tumor (3rd–4th decade)

Symptoms:
- Rapidly growing mass
- Severe pain
- Restriction of movement grossly

OSTEOSARCOMA

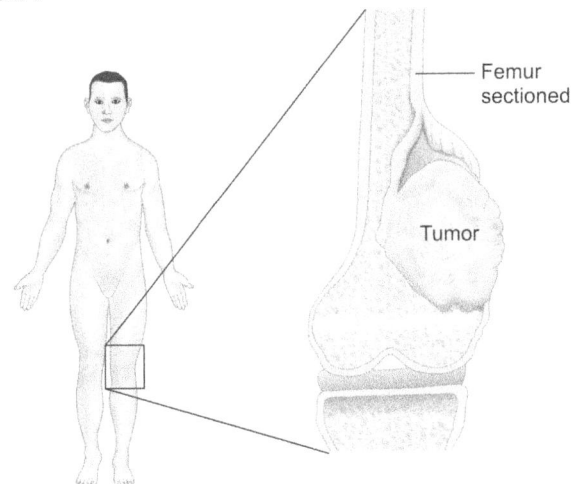

Q. Write clinical features, investigations and treatment of osteosarcoma.

Clinical features:

Symptoms:
- Age—2nd decade usual presentation
- Rapidly growing mass
- Origin—diaphysis
- Severe pain with huge swelling

Signs (common for all malignancy):
- Local tenderness
- Shiny skin
- Engorgement of veins with local venous prominence.
- Variegated feeling of the mass.

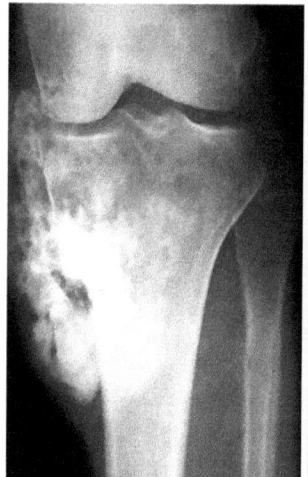
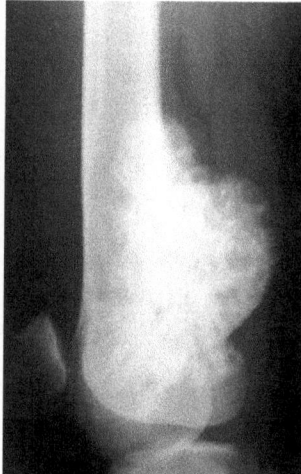

Investigaions:
- X-ray:
  - Differential diagnosis—osteosarcoma, Ewing's sarcoma, chondrosarcoma, chronic osteomyelitis for onion peel appearance.
  - Malignant tumor mass will never have discharge of pus, i.e., discharging sinus—it is a diagnostic sign of chronic osteomylelitis may get healed sinus.
- MRI: T2 signal followed by area of osteolysis, osteosclerosis and osteonecrosis.
- History and physical examination: Osteoid lined by malignant osteoblast +/− tumor giant cells. Formation of bone by the tumor cells are characteristic.

Treatment:
- After confirmation of diagnosis, chemotherapy should be started—vincristine, vinblastine, methotrexate, cyclophosphamide, etc.
- Reconstructive surgery followed by arthroplasty by custom made prosthesis or arthrodesis.
- Paliative surgery
- Amputation—one joint above the tumor location.
- Radiotherapy if necessary

Bone Tumors

EWING'S SARCOMA

Q Write clinical features, investigations and treatment of Ewing's sarcoma.

Clinical features:
- Origin: Metaphysis of long bone
- Common site: Around knee joint or pelvic bone
- Pain and sudden onset swelling, with severe tenderness.

Investigation:
- X-ray—periosteal reaction, onion peel appearance, Codmann's triangle.
- Pathology: History and physical examination—small round malignant tumor cell +/– rosette

Treatment
- Most radiosensitive (6,000–8,000 rads/per cycle) with combination of chemotherapy and palliative surgery.
- Reconstructive surgery followed by arthroplasty by custom-made prosthesis or arthrodesis.
- Amputation—one joint above the tumor location.

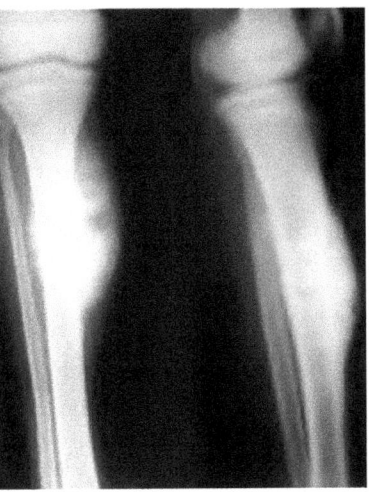

CHONDROSARCOMA

Q Write clinical feature, investigation, pathology, and treatment of chondrosarcoma.

Clinical features: Progressive swelling, pain around knee, local tenderness at joint line with restricted mobility, increased venous prominence.

Investigation:

X-ray:
- Cotton wool appearance (radiological)
- Chondrocytes are huge in number in history and physical examination.

MRI: Increased T2 signal

Pathology: History and physical examination—malignant chondrocytes, stromal cell.

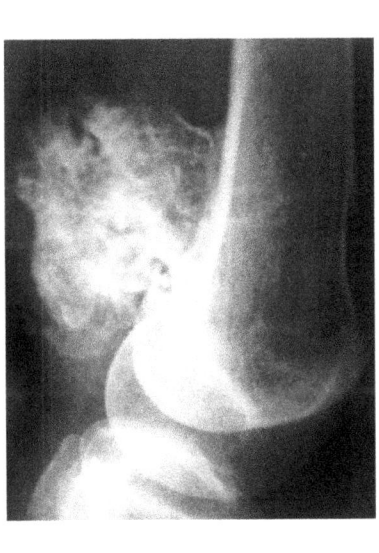

Treatment:
- After confirmation of diagnosis, chemotherapy should be started—vincristine, vinblastine, methotrexate, cyclophosphamide, etc.
- Radiotherapy sensitive, e.g., Ewing's sarcoma.
- Reconstructive surgery, followed by arthroplasty by custom made prosthesis or arthrodesis.
- Palliative surgery
- Amputation—one joint above the tumor location.

MULTIPLE MYELOMA

Q Write short notes on multiple myeloma.

- Most common primary malignant bone tumor
- Occur in elderly

Clinical features:

- Low backache, swelling over spine
- Kyphoscoliosis
- Multiple fracture at spine

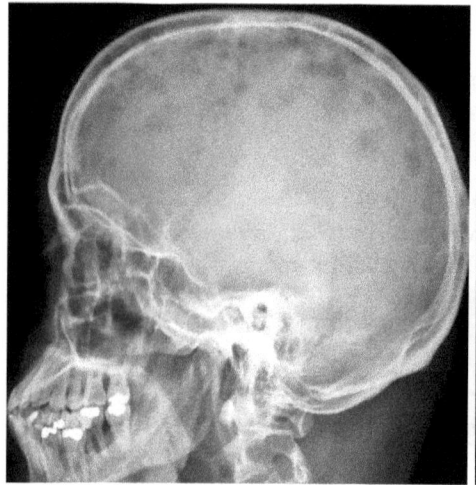
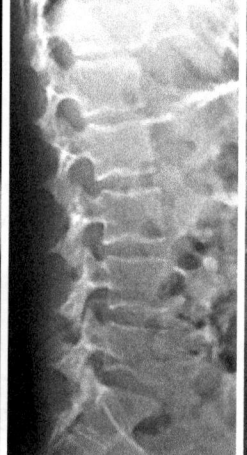
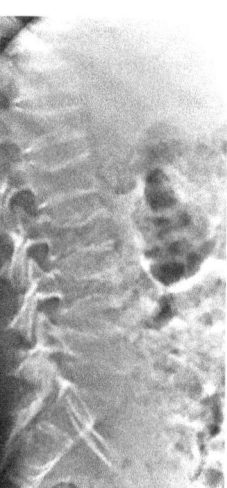

Skull X-ray—multiple punched out lesion   Spine—multiple compression fractures

Investigations:

- X-ray:
  - Spine—multiple compression fractures and decreased disc space
  - Skull—multiple punched out lesion
- Blood:
  - Erythrocyte sedimentation rate (ESR)—increased
  - Serum electrophoresis for M band (+ve)
- Urine: For Bence-Jones protein (+ve)
- MRI of spine: To detect cord compression
- History and physical examination: Sheets of malignant plasma cell.

Treatment:

- Rest
- Immobilization
- Nonsteroidal anti-inflammatory drugs (NSAIDs)
- Spinal brace (Boston's)
- Chemotherapy (vincristine, adriamycin, methotrexate)
- Surgery: Spinal stabilization by pedicle screw fixation

CHAPTER 9

Amputations

LOWER LIMB AND UPPER LIMB AMPUTATION

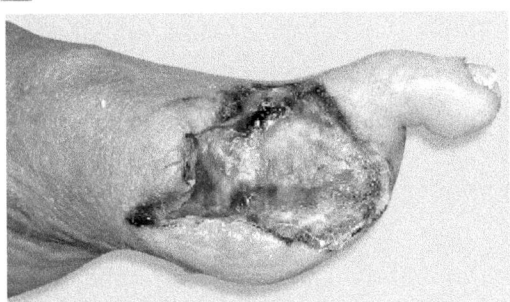 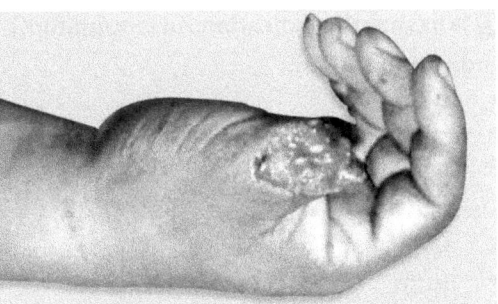

Q What are different types of lower limb amputations?
1. Hind quarter—pelvic bone is divided
2. Disarticulation of hip
3. Above knee
4. Below knee
5. Knee disarticulation
6. Syme's amputation
7. Partial foot amputation
8. Toe amputation.

Q Mention different types of upper limb amputation.
1. Fore-quarter amputation—at the level of scapula
2. Shoulder disarticulation
3. Above elbow
4. Bellow elbow
5. Elbow disarticulation
6. Wrist disarticulation
7. Amputation of fingers/digits

IDEAL AMPUTATION STUMP

Q What is an ideal amputation stump?
Ideal stump:

Types:
1. Definitive end-bearing (below knee/Syme's amputation)

2. Nonend-bearing (above or below elbow amputation)
    - Level should be distal to causal conditions
    - Sufficient cover of skin flap over deep tissue
    - The scar must not be terminal—for end-bearing
    - Bone end must be solid—for end-bearing
    - Bone must cut through or near a joint.

INDICATIONS OF AMPUTATION

Q What are the indications of amputation?

Indications (3D's):
1. Dead
2. Dangerous
3. Damn nuisance

Dead:
- Peripheral vascular disease (90%)
- Burns
- Crush injury in trauma
- Frostbite

Dangerous:
- Malignant tumor
- Gas gangrene
- Crush syndrome

Damn nuisance:
- Pain with gross malformation
- Recurrent sepsis
- Severe loss of function

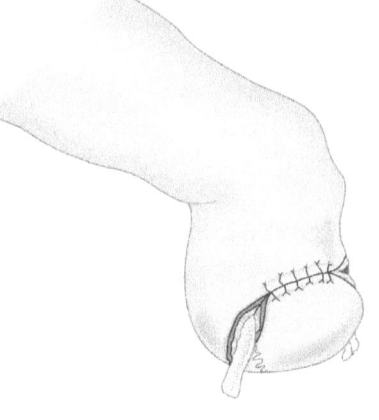

BELOW-KNEE AMPUTATIONS

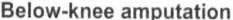
Below-knee amputation

Q Write short note on below-knee amputations.
- A healthy stump is well fitted with prosthesis will allow good range of function and near about normal gait.
- Stump should be 5–6 cm by length from knee joint.
- Adequate posterior skin flap to cover deep tissue.
- End-tibial and fibular bones should be adequately covered by posterior gastrosoleus muscles.
- Skin sutures should not be terminal.

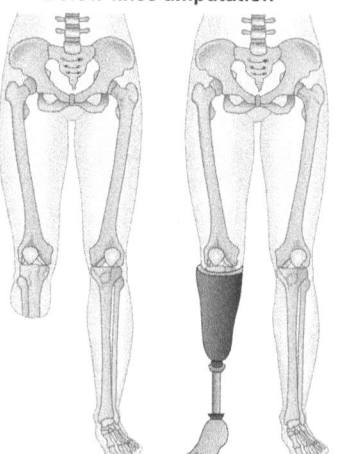

SYME'S AMPUTATION

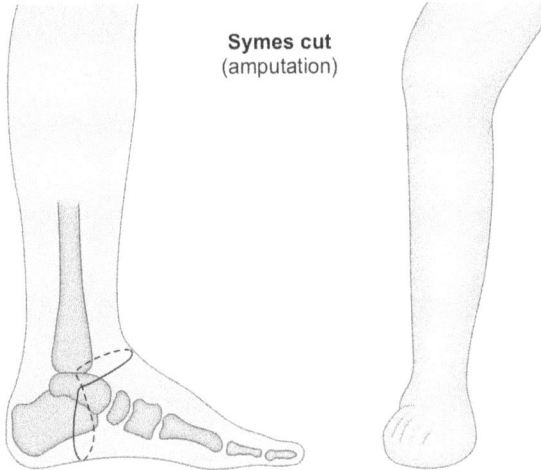

Symes cut (amputation)

Q What is Syme's amputation?
- The amputation level is above ankle.
- Indication—crush injury or functionless foot.
- The stump is end bearing
- The tibial and fibular bones are divided just above malleoli.
- Back to os calcis is stuck on cut end of tibia and fibula.
- Long posterior skin flap
- Flap contain skin with fibro-fatty tissue, to provide good pad for weight bearing.

CHAPTER 10

Sports Injury

KNEE INJURY

Q Describe knee injury.

Mechanism of injury:
- During football, rugby, hockey
- Younger age group

Symptoms:
- Huge knee swelling
- Sometimes could manage to walk. But do limping, squatting or unable to walk.
- Grossly restricted movement.

Signs:
- Tenderness at the affected area
- Whole tibio-femoral joint tenderness in anterior cruciate ligament (ACL)/anterior cruciate ligament (PCL) tear.

HEMARTHROSIS

Q Write short notes on hemarthrosis.
- Collection of blood in joint space
- In traumatic condition.
- Bleeding disorder
- Fracture of the femoral or tibial condyle, or patella, or fibula, etc.

Anterior cruciate ligament tear:

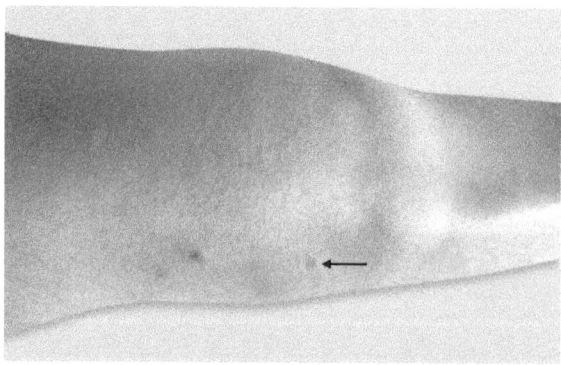

- Anterior drawer test—positive in ACL tear.
- Posterior drawer test—positive in PCL tear.
- Pivot test and Lachmann's test will be positive in ACL tear.

Meniscus injury: McMurray's test positive in medial and lateral meniscus, along with joint line tenderness accordingly.

Medial collateral (MCL) and lateral collateral (LCL) injury:
- Medial joint line is tender—in MCL injury
  - Varus test is positive—in MCL tear
  - Vulgus test is positive—in LCL tear

Investigations:
- X-ray of the affected limb to exclude the anterior tibial spine/posterior tibial spine fracture.
- Digital X-ray must be done in this case (anteroposterior/lateral/skyline view).
- Three-dimensional (3D) CT scan has a good role.
- MRI—clear-cut delineation of accurate injury
  - Grade I—partial tear
  - Grade II—partial tear
  - Grade III—complete tear
- Arthroscopy (diagnostic purpose), semi-invasive procedure.

Probable short note:
- Knee instability
- Hemarthosis
- Meniscus injury
- Cruciate injury
- Investigation in sports injury
- Arthroscopy

Treatment:
- Ice fomentation for reducing the swelling
- Nonsteroidal anti-inflammatory drugs (NSAIDs)—intramuscular (IM)/intravenous (IV)/oral
- Stabilization of the knee joint—strong immobilization by plaster slab/plaster of Paris (POP) cast [(above knee up to mid-thigh), below just above the ankle (cylindrical cast)]at 10–15° flexion of knee.
- Before immobilization—do the aspiration of the joint space only in the operation theater only, if there is huge swelling, otherwise not (functional position of hip—10° flexion, 5–10° external rotation, 10° abduction).

Operative:
- ACL tear/PCL tear: Arthroscopic ACL reconstruction by two way:
  - Patellar tendon bone graft (PTB graft)
  - Semitendinosus bone graft (semi-Td graft)
  - Semimembranosus graft
- MCL/LCT tear:
  - Do it as early as possible
  - Only suturing of the ligament

- Meniscus tear:
  - Suturing of meniscus by arthroscopy
  - Bucket handle tear—should think for meniscectomy may partial/complete.

KNEE LIGAMENT INJURIES

Q Describe knee ligament injuries.

Mechanism of injury:
- Direct by a dash board injury
- Indirect by combined rotation and impact (in a football tackle).

Clinical features:
- Pain, swelling, hemarthrosis
- Tenderness locally with range of movements of knee—grossly restricted.
- Anterior drawer test positive in anterior cruciate ligament injury.
- Posterior drawer test positive in posterior cruciate ligament injury.

McMurray's test—for meniscal injury:

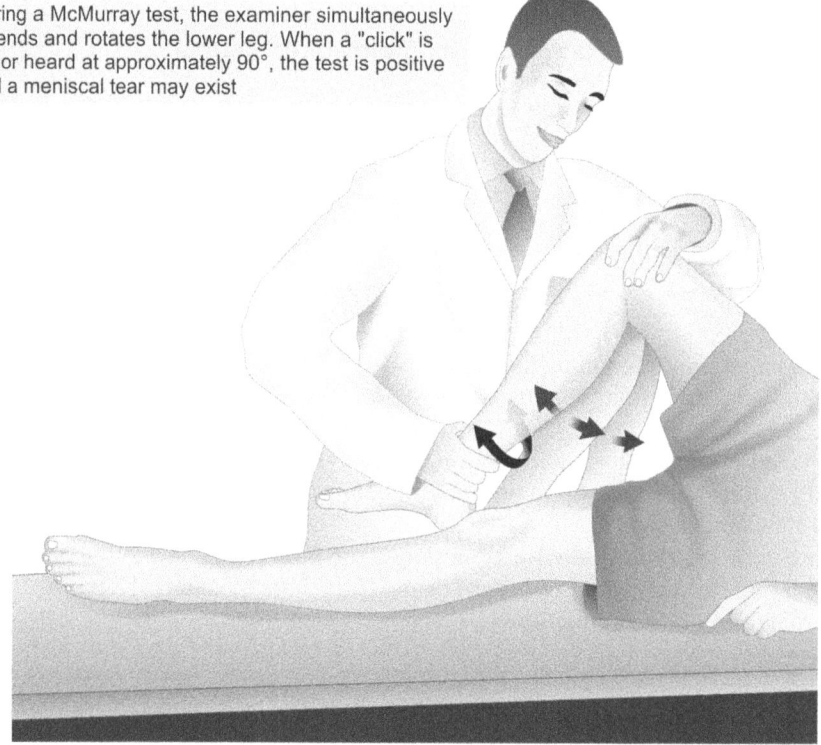

During a McMurray test, the examiner simultaneously extends and rotates the lower leg. When a "click" is felt or heard at approximately 90°, the test is positive and a meniscal tear may exist

- In supine position of patient
- By one hand surgeon palpate the medial and lateral joint line
- By other hand—surgeon will do forceful knee extension, when knee is flexed, abducted and externally rotated

- By this maneuver, patient will feel pain at affected side of meniscal injury and tenderness positive.

Investigation:
- X-ray of affected knee—anteroposterior and lateral view.
- MRI of affected knee

Treatment:
- In partial tears: Aspiration and above knee cylindrical POP cast for 6–8 weeks.
- In complete tears: Meniscectomy (partial/complete) or ACL/PCL reconstruction by bone patellar tendon graft (PTB) or semitendinosus tendon graft.

CHAPTER 11

Fractures

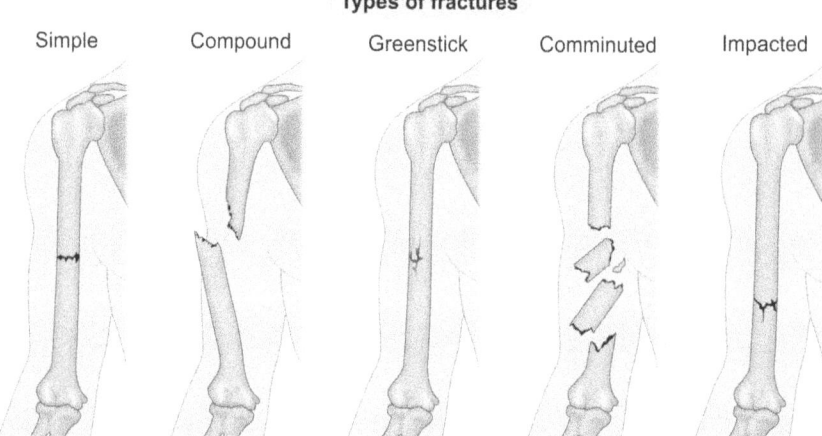

Types of fractures: Simple, Compound, Greenstick, Comminuted, Impacted

Q Define and classify fracture.

Fracture means breach in continuity of bone.

Classification:
1. According to displacement
    a. Undisplaced
    b. Displaced
2. According to wound
    a. Open—communicating outside skin
    b. Closed—no skin wound
3. According to fracture pattern
    a. Transverse
    b. Oblique
    c. Spiral
    d. Comminuted
    e. Segmental

STRESS FRACTURE

Q Write short notes on stress fracture.

- Fracture occurs in army personnel or sports injury, due to continuous stress on same site of bone.
- Usually undisplaced, unicortical break of bone and initially asymptomatic.

Clinical features: Gradually complaining of pain, swelling at fracture site with local tenderness ±, mild or no restriction of nearby joint movement.

Investigation:
- X-ray—may be missed initially as its mostly undisplaced cortical break
- CT scan—diagnostic
- Bone scan—will give the diagnosis

Treatment:
- Rest
- Immediate immobilization by plaster of Paris (POP) in fracture of long bone.
- If fracture nearby joint or deformity present—closed reduction and percutaneous pinning under image guide.

PATHOLOGICAL FRACTURE

Q Write short notes on pathological fracture.

Fracture occurs due to any pathological condition like:
- Osteoporosis
- Metastasis
- Bone tumors
- Rheumatoid arthritis
- Acute/chronic osteomyelitis
- Osteogenesis imperfecta

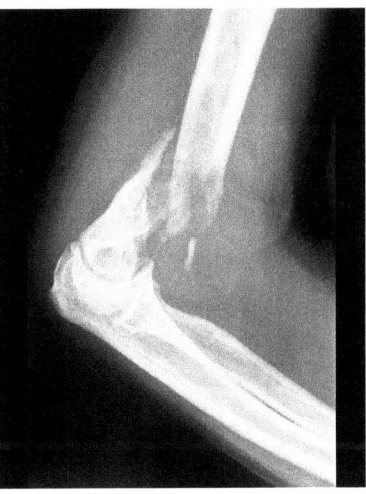

Clinical features:
- May be asymptomatic initially
- Low-grade pain, swelling
- Deformity
- Restricted movement gradually

Investigation:
- X-ray of local part
- Search of primary pathology
- Bone scan (whole body)
- MRI of affected area
- Urine for Bence-Jone's protein
- Serum electrophoresis
- Vitamin D_3 level estimations.

Treatment:
- Of primary pathology and reduction of fracture by open or closed means and internal fixation by interlocking nail/limited contact dynamic compression plate (LCDCP) or locking compression plate (LCP).
- If fracture near to a joint: Replacement arthroplasty can be done [total hip replacement (THR)/total knee replacement (TKR)/total elbow replacement (TER)].

OPEN (COMPOUND) FRACTURE

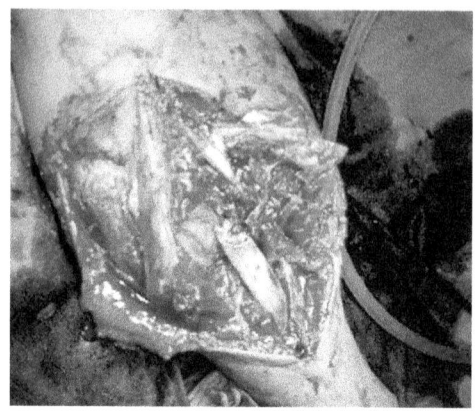

Q Define, classify and investigation of open fracture.

Here, the fracture is communicating with exterior through a wound.

Classification: According to Gustilo–Anderson

Types	Wound size	Velocity of trauma	Contamination	Bone exposed
Grade I	<1 cm	Low	Nil/Mild	No
Grade II	1–10 cm	Moderate	Moderate	No
Grade III	>10 cm	High	Severe	Yes, but covered by muscles
				No muscle cover
				Neurovascular injury

Investigation:

- Stabilize the patient hemodynamically by in vitro fertilization (IVF)/O_2 inhalation
- Rule out any other system injury.
- Thorough lavage of wound by normal saline (NS)—10-15 liter
- Adequate debridement
- Fixation of fracture by external/internal means.

EXTERNAL FIXATION

Q Write short notes on external fixation.

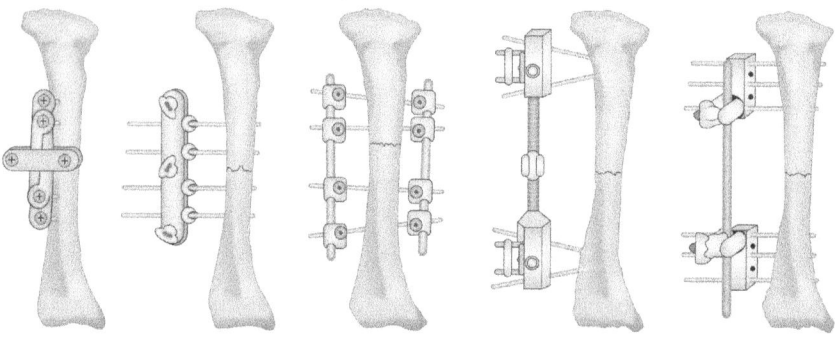

Indications:
- Open fracture
- Infected nonunion
- Limb lengthening

Implants used:
- Schanz pins
- Universal clamp
- Tubular rod
- T-clamp
- Tube to tube clamp

Types:
- Tubular fixator
- Ring fixator (Ilizarov)

Procedure for tubular fixator:
- Usually two parallel Schanz pins put each side of fracture—2 cm away from fracture, after drilling bone.
- Then assembly completed with universal clamp and connected through a AO tubular rod.
- T-clamp is necessary—if Fracture is nearby to a joint.

Procedure ring fixator:
- Usually 3–4 (360°) rings are put
- Stabilized by 2 k-wires/or (1 olive wire/1 k-wire) with a ring.
- All rings are stabilized by connecting rods.
- Corticotomy done at metaphyseal site, between two rings and will cause distraction.
- Other two rings are for compressing the fracture and for limb lengthening.

GREEN STICK FRACTURE

Q Write short notes on green stick fractures.

It is undisplaced fracture, occur in child.

Clinical features: Pain, swelling, restricted range of motion (ROM) of joint with deformity.

X-ray:
- Shows cortical contact is maintained but anterior or posterior bend is present.
- No rotational bend
- Sometimes unicortical break also there.

Treatment: Closed reduction, reduced under GA + immobilization by plaster of Paris (POP) cast or percutaneous pin under image guidance.

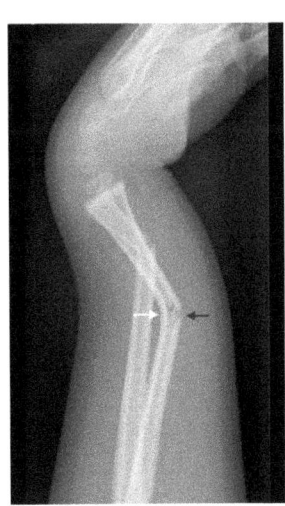

CHAPTER 12
Fractures Around Hip Joint

Fractures around hip joint are as follows:
1. Fracture neck of femur
2. Fracture intertrochanteric femur
3. Fracture subtrochanteric femur
4. Fracture head of femur
5. Fracture acetabulum
6. Fracture pelvis

FRACTURE NECK OF FEMUR

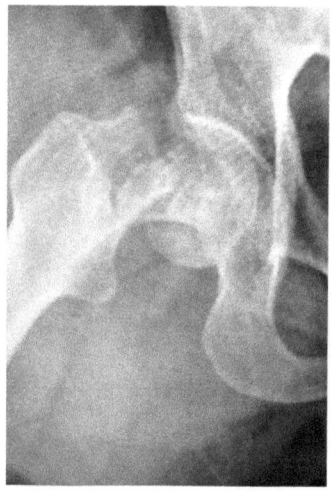
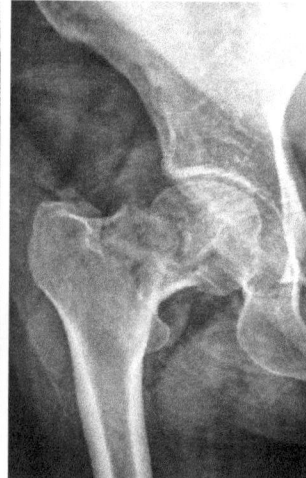
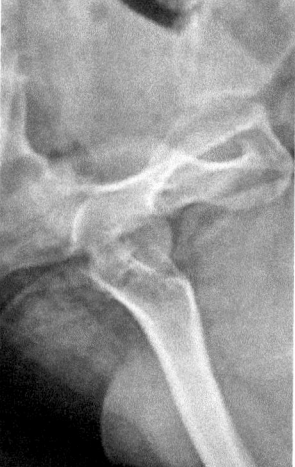

Q Describe clinical features, classification, and treatment fracture of neck of femur and its complication.

Mechanism of injury:
- In child, renal tubular acidosis (RTA)
- In aged person (>60 years) following trivial trauma.

Clinical features:

Symptoms:
- Pain (main complaint)
- Swelling—nothing
- Range of movements—grossly restricted
- Difficulty in standing/walking.

Signs:
- Local tenderness, at anterior point of hip joint.
- Straight leg rising (SLR)—patient can do SLR in normal but in fracture neck of femur (NOF)—there is no SLR.
- Range of movement.
  - Flexion
  - Extension
  - Abduction ⎫
  - Adduction ⎬—All restricted in painful
  - Rotation (internal)
  - Rotation (external) ⎭

Investigation:
- X-ray pelvis with both hip joint (anteroposterior view)
- Affected hip with thigh (lateral view)

Classification:
1. Anatomical classification—by X-ray
   - Subcapital
   - Transcervical
   - Basicervical
2. Pauel's classification:

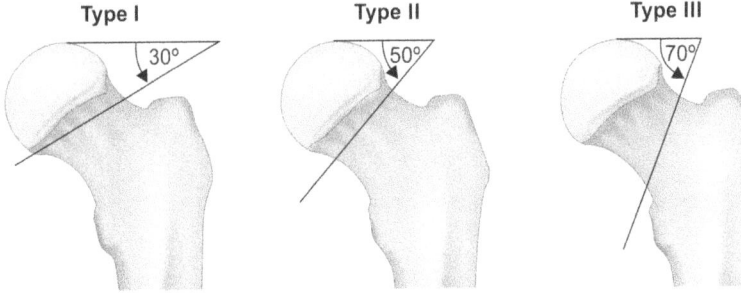

   - Type I: 30–50°
   - Type II: 50–70°
   - Type III: >70°
3. Garden's classification:

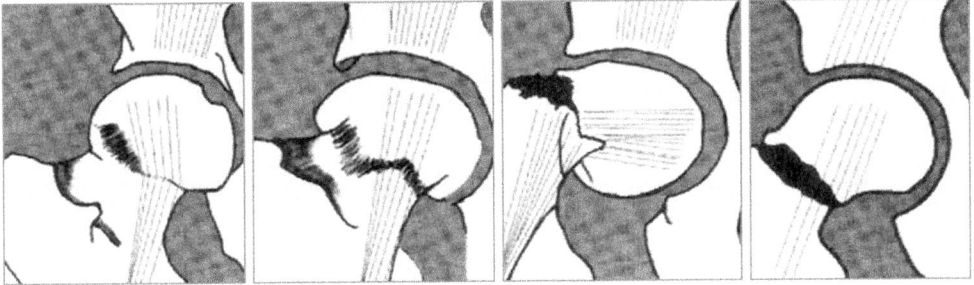

- Grade I: Impacted, incomplete, undisplaced.
- Grade II: Complete, undisplaced.
- Grade III: Complete, displaced fracture and acetabular trabeculae and proximal femoral trabeculae are not in same line.
- Grade IV: Complete fracture, displaced and rotated completely so that acetabular trabeculae and proximal femoral trabeculae are in same line.

Treatment:
- *For child:* Closed reduction and internal fixation with percutaneous pinning (K-wire, Knowle's pin).
- *For adult (<60 years):* Closed reduction and internal fixation with cannulated cancellous hip screw (CHS) under image intensifier.
- *For old patient (>60 years):* Hemiarthroplasty (unipolar, bipolar) and total hip replacement (THR).

Complication:

Nonunion (most common) follow by:
- Malunion
- Avascular necrosis
- Joint stiffness
- Secondary osteoarthritis

INTERTROCHANTERIC FRACTURE

Q Define clinical features, investigation, classification and treatment of intertrochanteric fracture.

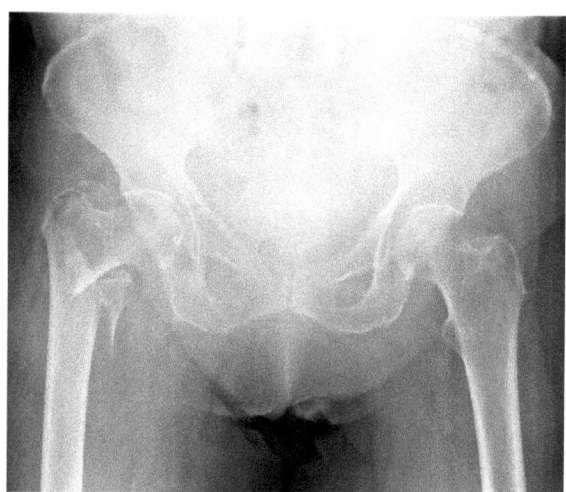

Mechanism of injury
- Trivial trauma
- Renal tubular acidosis (RTA)

Symptoms:
- Same as before

- Swelling around hip
- Bruise and echymosis around trochanter.

Signs:
- Local tenderness in intertrochanteric region
- Straight leg rising (positive)

Classification (Boyd and Griffin's):
- Undisplaced
- Minimally displaced
- Displaced and rotated

Treatment: It can be managed by conservative treatment by skeletal traction and/or closed reduction and internal fixation (CRIF) with dynamic hip screw (DHS) with 135° barrel plate with screws.

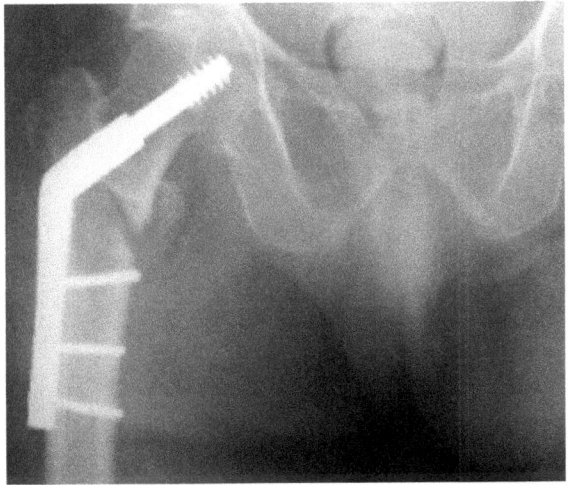

SUBTROCHANTERIC FRACTURE

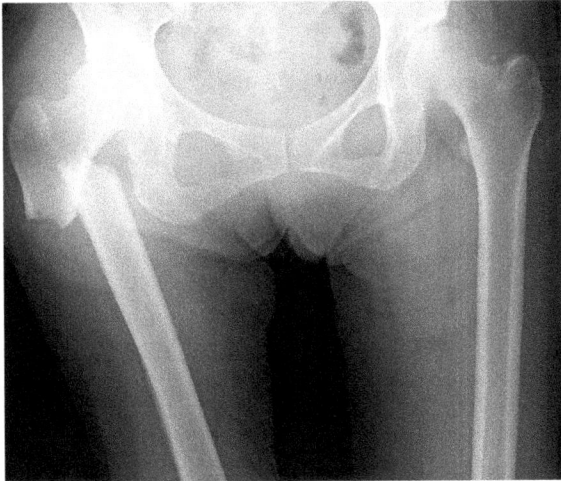

Q Fracture level is below lesser trochanter.
Clinical features, investigations, and treatment—same as intertrochanteric fracture.

Q Describe clinical features, investigation and treatment of subtrochanteric fracture.

Symptoms:
- Pain (main complaint)
- Swelling—nothing
- Range of movements—grossly restricted
- Difficulty in standing/walking.

Signs:
- Local tenderness, below trochanteric region.
- Straight leg rising (SLR)—there is no SLR.
- Range of movement.
  - Flexion
  - Extension
  - Abduction — All restricted in painful
  - Adduction
  - Rotation (internal)
  - Rotation (external)

Investigation:
- X-ray pelvis with both hip joint (anteroposterior view)
- Affected hip with thigh (lateral view)

Treatment:
- Can be managed by conservative treatment by skeletal traction and/or closed reduction and internal fixation (CRIF) with dynamic hip screw (DHS) with 135° barrel plate with screws, under image guidance.
- Can be treated by closed reduction and internal fixation by proximal femoral nail (PFN) under image guidance.

FRACTURE HEAD OF FEMUR

Clinical features: All are same, like intertrochanteric fracture.

Classification: Pipkin's classification (Grade I–V)

Investigation:
- Computed tomography (CT) scan and X-ray
- Three-dimensional (3D) CT scan
- Magnetic resonance imaging (MRI)

Treatment:
- Patient is usually young adult—open reduction and internal fixation by headless cancellous screw.
- If fracture is large—hemiarthroplasty

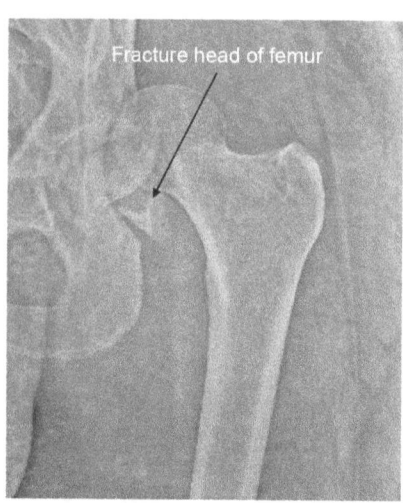
Fracture head of femur

Complications:
- Nonunion followed by malunion
- Avascular necrosis of femoral head
- Stiff hip

ACETABULAR FRACTURE

Q Describe mechanism of injury, investigation, treatment, and complication of fracture head of femur.

Mechanism of injury:
- Very common in RTA
- Symptoms and signs are same
- Some patient can do SLR (not always)

Investigation: X-ray of pelvis both hip (anteroposterior view), internal oblique and external oblique view.

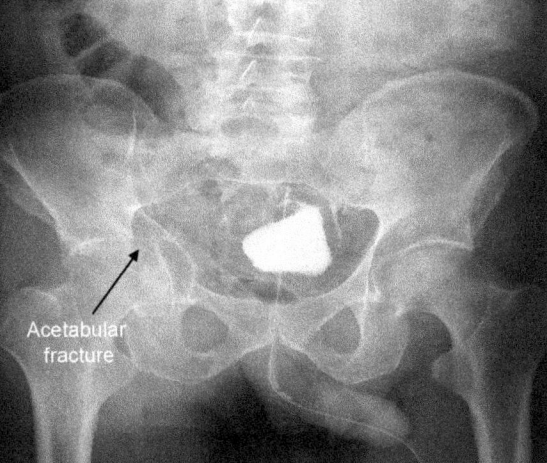
Acetabular fracture

Treatment:
- Open reduction and internal fixation by reconstruction plate with cancellous screw according to the shape of the acetabulum and fracture anatomy.
- Total hip replacement (THR) in old fracture acetabulum.

Complication:
- Sciatic nerve palsy
- Secondary osteoarthritis hip
- Stiff hip joint

FRACTURE PELVIS

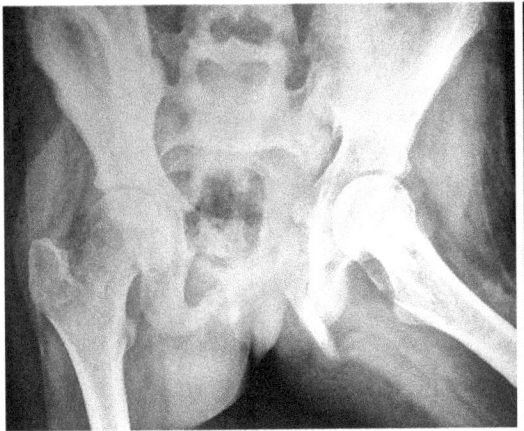
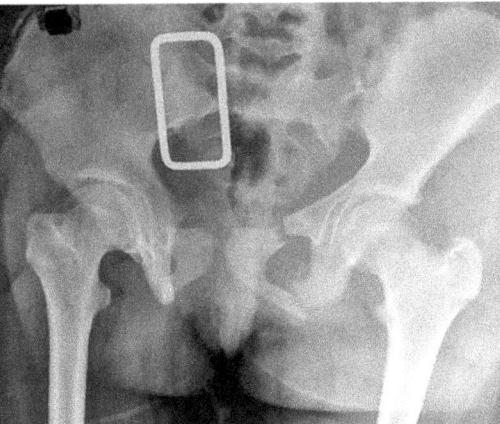

Q. Describe classification, investigation, and treatment of fracture pelvis.

Mechanism of injury:
- High velocity trauma—mainly RTA
- Fall from multistoried building.

Classification (Tile's):
1. Stable
2. Rotationally unstable but vertically stable
3. Unstable in all way—both rotationally and vertically.

Investigation:
- X-ray (anteroposterior, lateral, internal and external iliac view)
- CT scan must, USG abdomen

Treatment:
- Management of shock by 2–3 units blood transfusion—must
- Pelvic binder or brace tightly
- Rule out any visceral injury
- If unstable fracture—closed reduction and external fixation under image guidance in emergency as life-saving measure and repair of visceral injury with utmost care.
- When the patient is hemodynamically stable—will be treated by open reduction and internal fixation by reconstruction plate and cancellous screw.

CHAPTER 13: Fracture Around Knee and Above

FRACTURE PATELLA

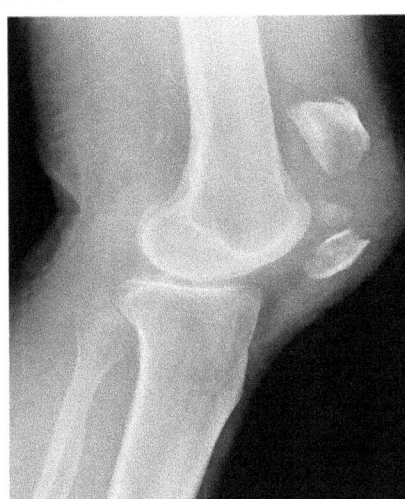 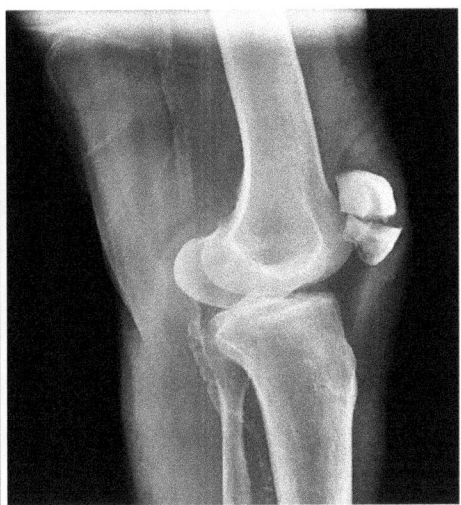

Q Define clinical features, investigations, and treatment of fracture patella.

Mechanism of injury:
- Direct force—fall/or blow against dashboard of car.
- Indirect—if foot caught against a solid obstacle.

Clinical features:
- Pain, swelling at anterior part of knee
- Abrasion, bruise over the joint
- Tenderness +ve over patella
- Palpable gap—if grossly displaced
- Hemarthrosis

Investigation:
- X-ray of affected knee (anteroposterior and lateral view)
- CT scan—to rule out any intra-articular fragments, if not clearly visible by X-ray.

Treatment:
- For undisplaced fracture: Above knee cylindrical plaster of Paris (POP) cast for 4 weeks.
- For displaced fracture: Open reduction + internal fixation by tension band wiring (TBW).

TENSION BAND WIRING

Q Write short note on tension band wiring.

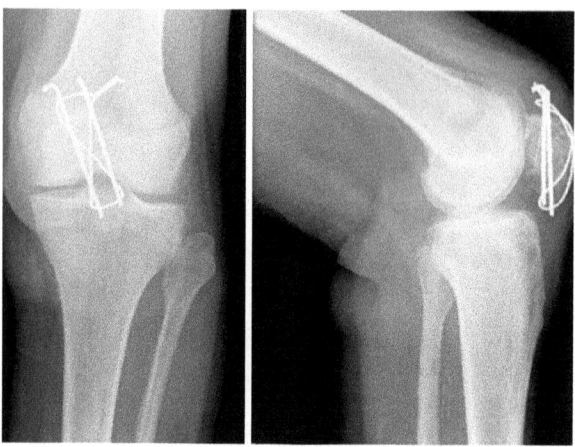

Principle: Converts tensile force into compressible force.

Method:
- Anterior midline incision to knee
- Medial parapatellar approach
- Fracture fragment exposed and reduced by open means
- Hold by patellar holding clamp
- Pass two parallel K-wire from above downward and one S-S wire passed through uuadriceps tendon above and patellar ligament bellow, in 'figure of 8' manner, which will cause— compression at fracture site and wound closed in layers.

FRACTURE FEMORAL CONDYLE

Q Write clinical feature, investigation and treatment of fracture femoral condyle.

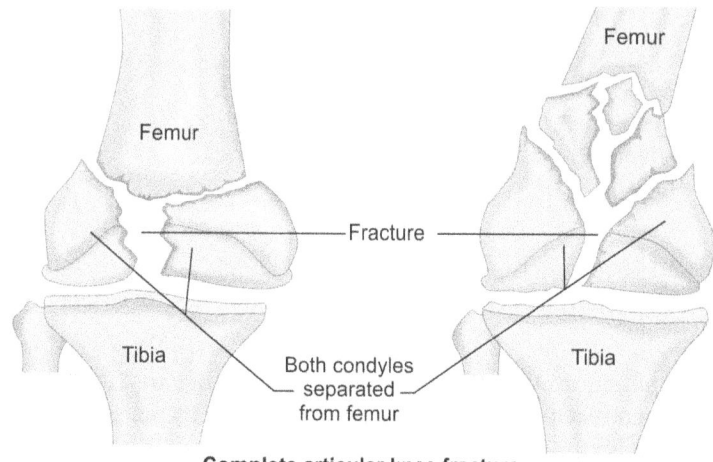

Complete articular knee fracture

Fracture Around Knee and Above

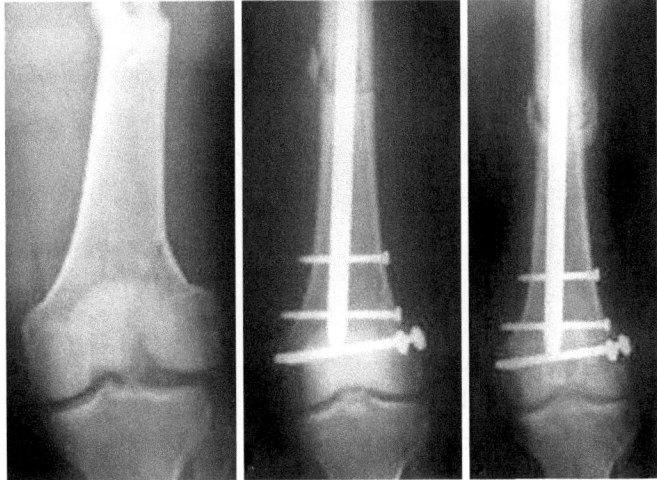

Mechanism of injury:
- Direct injury—in RTA
- Indirect—fall from height

Clinical features:
- Pain, swelling around knee
- Tenderness +ve
- Range of movements—grossly restricted
- Hemarthrosis

Investigation:
- X-ray of knee and thigh (anteroposterior and lateral view)
- CT scan
- MRI of knee—to detect intra-articular fragment

Treatment:
- Open reduction and internal fixation by cancellous screw
- Dynamic condylar screw (DCS) with condylar plate and screw under image guidance.

TIBIAL PLATEAU FRACTURE OR FRACTURE OF TIBIAL CONDYLE

Q How will you manage a case of tibial plateau fracture or fracture of tibial condyle and describe its complications?

Mechanism of injury:
- Direct—by car striking a pedestrian
- Indirect—by fall from height

Clinical features:
- Pain, swelling around knee
- Hemarthrosis

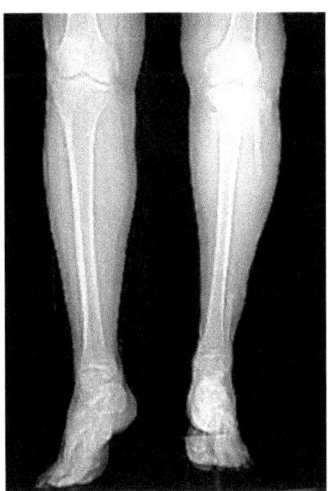

- Tenderness +ve
- Range of movements—grossly restricted
- May be associated with neurovascular injury—may lead to compartment syndrome.

Investigation:
- X-ray of knee with leg (anteroposterior and lateral view)
- CT scan
- MRI of knee
- If vascular status doubtful:
  - Doppler study or
  - Angiography

Classification (Schatzkar classification—six types):

Type I: Undisplaced fracture lateral condyle

Type II: Comminuted fracture lateral condyle with depression

Type III: Comminuted, depressed with intact lateral fragment

Type IV: Fracture medial condyle

Type V: Fracture both condyles

Type VI: Combined condylar and subcondylar fracture

Treatment:
- Open reduction and internal fixation by cancellous screw (type I)
- Lateral buttress plate + screw in types II and III
- Medial buttress plate and screw in type IV
- Bicondylar plate in types V and VI

Complication of any fracture around knee:
- Joint stiffness
- Valgus or varus deformity
- Osteoarthritis (OA) of knee
- In tibial plateau fracture: Neurovascular injury is the most dreadful immediate complication leads to compartment syndrome and followed by gangrene in neglected cases.

KNEE DISLOCATION

Q Write short notes on knee dislocation.

Mechanism of injury: Commonly by high velocity trauma in road accident.

Clinical features:
- Swelling, pain gross deformity

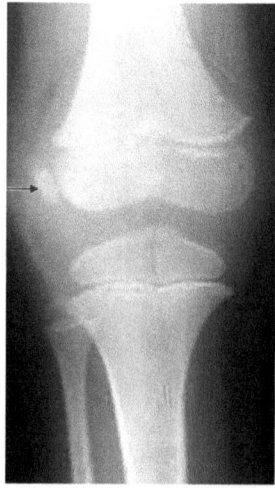
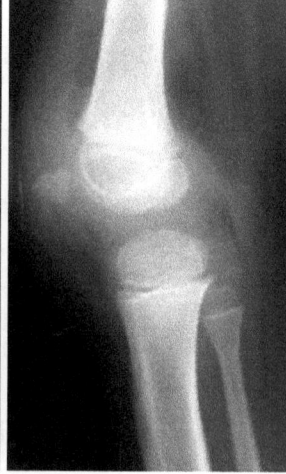

- Severe bruise, abrasions, hemarthrosis
- Neurovascular injury occur commonly—distal pulse/sensation should be tested (chance of popliteal vessel injury).

Investigation:
- X-ray of knee (anteroposterior and lateral view)
- Color Doppler study
- MRI of knee

Treatment:
- Under anesthesia: Closed reduction + splintage on *Bohler Braun* (BB) splint by skeletal traction (lower tibial) for 10–15 days.
- When anterior knee swelling subsides cylindrical POP cast for 6 weeks.

FRACTURE SHAFT OF FEMUR

Q Describe mechanism of injury, clinical features, investigation and treatment of fracture shaft of femur.

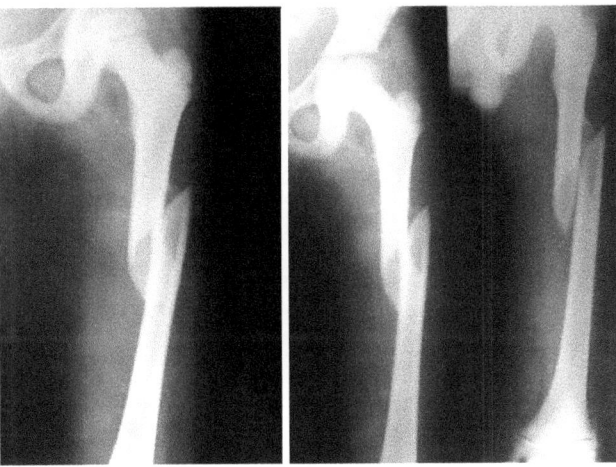

Mechanism of injury:
- Indirect—by fall with twisting force
- Direct—violence cause transverse/oblique fracture

Clinical Features:
- Usually young adults with severe shock
- Leg is short, deformed and externally rotated
- Thigh is swollen, tender with bruise.
- Fat embolism—with respiratory distress is common [acute respiratory distress syndrome (ARDS)] and petechial hemorrhagic spot throughout body (in urine examination—fat globules present).

Investigation:
- X-ray of affected thigh (anteroposterior and lateral view)

- X-ray of hip/knee—anteroposterior and lateral view (is must) to rule of fracture neck of femur/patella fracture.
- Urine of fat globules—in fat embolism present.

Treatment:
- Correction of shock
- Blood transfusion
- Splintage of limb with skeletal traction
- Closed reduction + internal fixation (CRIF) by interlocking nail (ILN) or open reduction + internal fixation (ORIF) by K-nail/dynamic compression plate (DCP)/limited contact dynamic compression plate (LCDCP).

CHAPTER 14: Fracture Around Ankle and Above

FRACTURE OF TIBIA

Mechanism of injury:
- Direct blow in motor cycle accidents
- Indirect twisting of leg

Q Describe clinical features, classification, investigation and treatment of fracture both bone (# BB) of leg.

Clinical features:
- Pain, swelling deformity of leg
- Tenderness +ve
- Leg may be bruised with abrasions
- May be open fracture—fracture is communicating with exteriors.

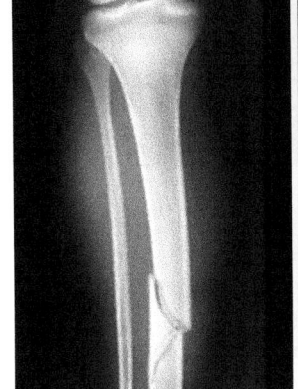
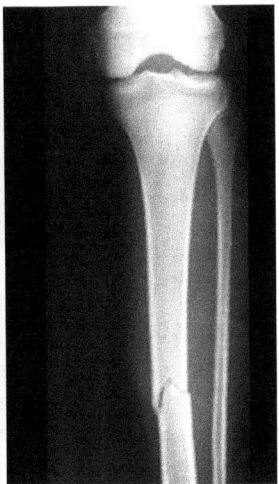

Gustilo-Anderson classification of open fracture:

Three types:

Type I: Wound size <1 cm, no contamination, low velocity traumas.

Type II: Wound size 1–10 cm, moderate contamination, moderate velocity trauma.

Type III: Wound size >10 cm, severe contamination, high velocity trauma.

Three subtypes:

Type A: Fracture bone is not exposed outside skin.

Type B: Fracture bone exposed outside skin.

Type C: Associated first neurovascular injury and crush injury.

Investigations:
- X-ray of leg—anteroposterior and lateral view
- Color Doppler study—in type III open fracture
- Angiography—in type III C open fracture

Treatment:
- In closed fracture: Undisplaced (anterior knee)—plaster of Paris (POP) cast for 8 weeks.
- In displaced fracture: Closed reduction + internal fixation by interlocking nail or open reduction + internal fixation with V-nail/limited contact dynamic compression plate (LCDCP).

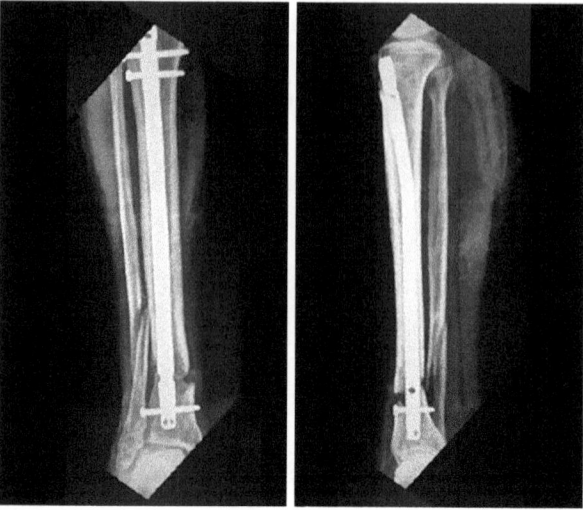

In open fracture

It is managed by:
- Wound lavage and debridement
- Stabilization by external fixators

(Put two Schanz pins above and two pins bellow fracture and make an assembly by four universal clamps and one AO tubular rod)

FRACTURE MEDIAL MALLEOLI AND FRACTURE LATERAL MALLEOLI

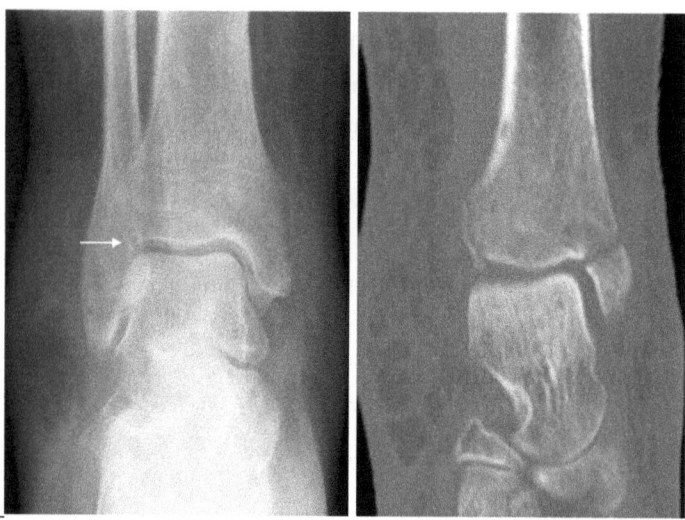

Mechanism of injury: Twisting force to ankle mortise (mainly talus) along with external rotation with abduction/adduction.

Q Describe clinical features, investigation, and treatment of trimalleolar fracture.

Clinical features:
- Swelling, pain at affected ankle
- Local tenderness:
  - If fracture medial malleoli—medial tenderness
  - If fracture lateral malleoli—lateral tenderness
- Range of movements of ankle—grossly restricted

Investigation: X-ray of ankle—anteroposterior, lateral and mortise view (1/2 oblique).

Treatment:
- If undisplaced fracture: Closed reduction + percutaneous pin under image guidance.
- If displaced fracture: Open reduction and internal fixation by malleolar screw or tension band wiring (TBW) for fracture medial malleoli.
- Fracture lateral malleoli: Open reduction (OR) + internal fixation (IF) by 1/3 semitubular plate and screw.
- Fracture of posterior malleoli: OR + IF with malleolar screw.

FRACTURE TALUS

Q Mention clinical features, investigation and treatment of fracture talus.

Mechanism of injury: By car accident or fall from height.

Clinical features:
- Swelling, deformed ankle
- Skin may be split or necrose
- Arteria dorsalis pedis should be palpable

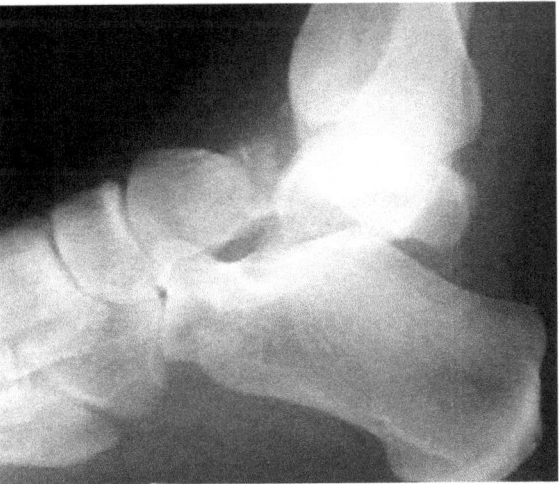

Investigation: X-ray ankle (anteroposterior, lateral and oblique view).

Treatment:
- Undisplaced fracture: Bellow knee POP cast for 8 weeks
- Displaced fracture: OR + IF with lag screw (on urgent basis) + limb elevation
- If swelling decreases—then (BK) POP splint for 3 weeks and (BK) POP cast for 6 weeks.

FRACTURE CALCANEUM

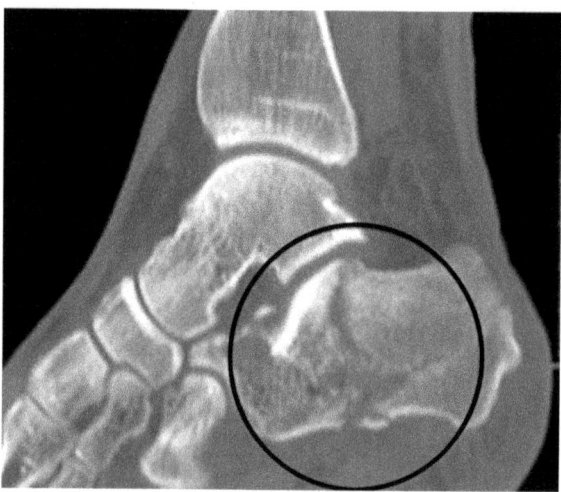

Q Describe mechanism of injury, clinical features, investigation, and treatment of fracture calcaneum.

Mechanism of injury: Fall from height—same accident may cause injury to spine, pelvis/hip also.

Clinical features:
- Swelling, painful foot
- Bruise over sole
- Range of ankle—impossible
- Normal concavity below lateral malleoli is lacking.

Investigation: X-ray of foot—(anteroposterior, lateral and oblique view).

Treatment:
- Elevation of leg and foot and ice application
- For extra-articular fracture—bellow knee POP cast for 6 weeks.
- For intra-articular fracture—open reduction with internal fixation (ORIF) with H-plate or Y-plate + cancellous screw under image guidance.

FRACTURE TARSAL BONES

Treatment: Open reduction and internal fixation by cancellous screw if fracture is displaced (if undisplaced fracture—below knee POP cast for 4 weeks).

FRACTURE METATARSAL BONES OR FRACTURE PHALANX

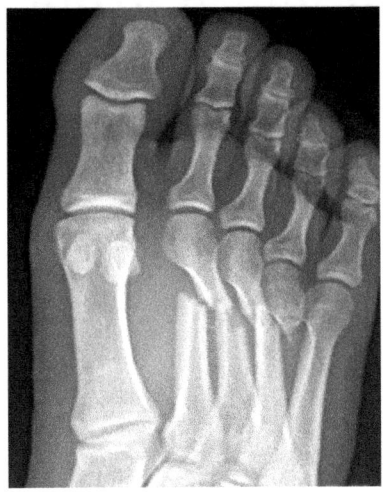

Treatment:
- If undisplaced fracture: Below knee POP cast for 4 weeks
- If displaced fracture: ORIF with K-wire/small LCDCP with screw or CRIF with K-wire/titanium elastic nail system (TENS) under image.

CHAPTER 15

Fracture Around Shoulder

Q Mention fractures occurring due to fall in outstretched hand.
- Fracture supracondylar humerus
- Fracture lateral condyle
- Fracture medial condyle
- Fracture (intra-articular) distal humerus
- Monteggia fracture dislocation
- Galeazzi fracture dislocation
- Colles' fracture
- Smith fracture
- Fracture clavicle

FRACTURE CLAVICLE

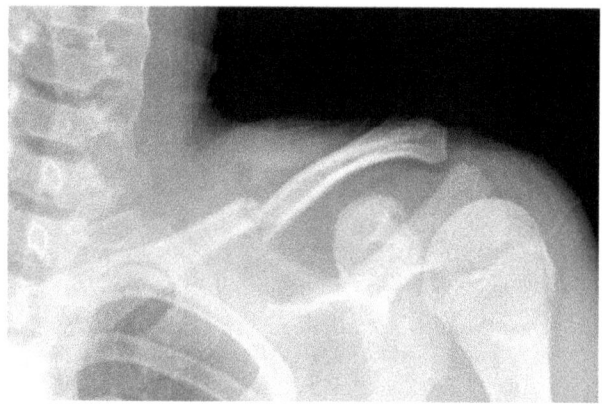

Mechanism of injury: Fall on outstretched hand or direct fall in shoulder.

Q How will you manage a case of clinical features?

Clinical features:

Subcutaneous lump, pain, or projected fracture fragment through skin.
Restricted shoulder range of movements.

Investigation:

X-ray:
- Usually occur in M/3 of bone.
- But may be outer 1/3 also.

Treatment:
- Closed reduction + figure of '8' bandage or clavicular brace and arm sling.
- If grossly displaced fracture: Open reduction + internal fixation by reconstruction plate and screws or clavicular plate and screws.

Complication:
- Nonunion
- Malunion
- Stiffness of shoulder
- Subclavian artery injury (immediate)

DISLOCATION OF SHOULDER

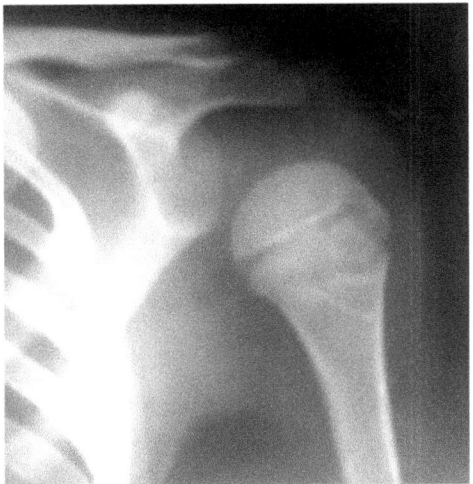

Q Mention classification, clinical features, investigation and treatment of dislocation of shoulder.

Types: Anterior (98%) and posterior (2%)
- Anterior dislocation: Most common inferomedial
- Mechanism: Fall on outstretched hand

Clinical features:
- Severe pain
- Swelling on anterior shoulder
- Patient supports arm by opposite hand
- Hamilton Ruler's test +ve, and Duga's test +ve

Investigation:
- X-ray—overlapping shadow of head (glenoid usually lying below and medial).
- Hill Sac's sign—flattening of part of lateral corner of humeral head.

Treatment:
- Closed reduction under general anesthesia (GA) + arm chest bandage for 1 month.

- Rest of arm in a sling.
- Physiotherapy of elbow/fingers.

Complication:
- Early: Neurovascular injury—rest
- Late:
    - Shoulder stiffness
    - Unreduced dislocation
    - Recurrent dislocation

RECURRENT DISLOCATION OF SHOULDER

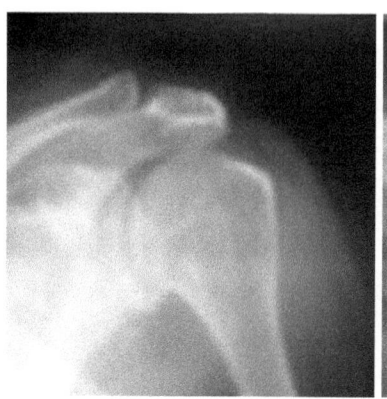
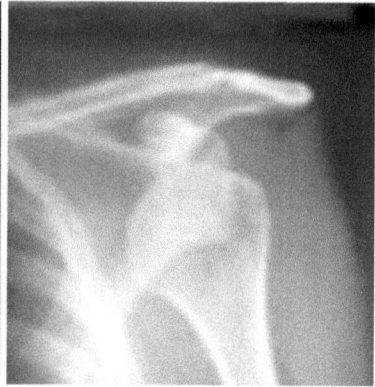

Q Write definition, clinical features, investigation, and treatment of recurrent dislocation.

Head of humerus comes out of socket, frequently at least >3 times, due to stress activity and patient himself may relocate.

Clinical features: Mild pain, swelling, fovea of dislocation in extreme external rotation and abduction.

Investigation: MRI—shows capsular tear with Bankart's lesion and Hill Sach's lesion.

Treatment:
- Bankart's procedure
- Bristow procedure—reconstruction of coracoid process through capsule
- Putti-Platt procedure—double breasting of shoulder capsule.

FRACTURE NECK OF HUMERUS

Mechanism of injury: Fall in outstretched hand.

Clinical features:
- Pain, swelling at shoulder

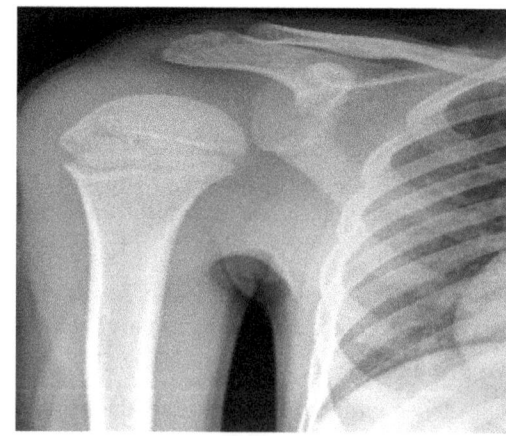

- Tenderness positive at the shoulder joint line.
- Range of movements of shoulder restricted.

X-ray of shoulder (anteroposterior and axial view)—fracture seen.

Classification of fracture neck of humerus—Neer's classification (Type I to VI):

Type I: Undisplaced
Type II: One part fracture
Type III: Two part fracture
Type IV: Three part fracture
Type V: Four part or more or comminuted fracture
Type VI: Type V with dislocation

Treatment:
- If undisplaced fracture immobilization by POP cast (U cast) or
- If displaced fracture—ORIF/CRIF by locking plate (LCP)/or PHILOS.

FRACTURE SHAFT OF HUMERUS

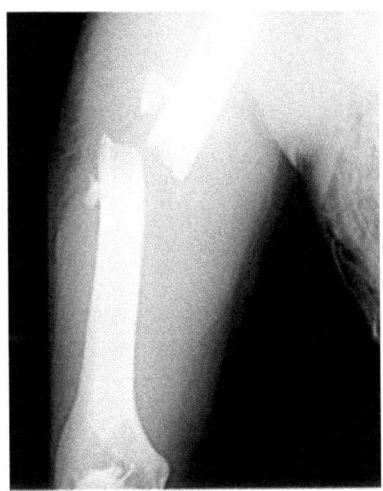

Mechanism of injury: Fall in outstretched hand.

Clinical features:
- Pain, swelling at fracture site of arm
- Range of movements of shoulder/elbow—restricted.

X-ray: Fracture seen.

Treatment: Closed reduction + immobilization by POP cast (U cast) or interlocking nail under image guidance/or limited contact DCP plate (LCDCP).

CHAPTER 16: Fracture Around Elbow Joint

Types of fracture around elbow are as follows:
1. Supracondylar fracture humerus
2. Intercondylar fracture humerus
3. Lateral condyle fracture humerus
4. Medial condyle fracture humerus
5. Head of radius
6. Fracture olecranon

SUPRACONDYLAR FRACTURE HUMERUS (EXTRA-ARTICULAR)

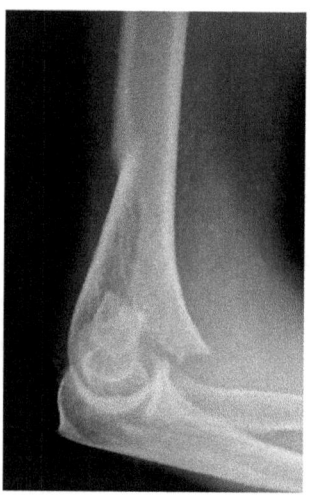

Q Describe mechanism, clinical features, of supracondylar fracture humerus.

Mechanism of injury:
- Outstretched hand fall
- Direct blow (2–5%)

Clinical features:

Symptoms: Swelling, pain, restriction of movement—inability to move elbow.

Signs:
- Local tenderness above the elbow
- Crepitus at the same side
- Compartment syndrome

Fracture Around Elbow Joint

Q Write short notes on compartment syndrome.

Compartment syndrome (both the compartments of forearm are tense):
- Complain of severe pain, swelling
- Fingers are swollen, tenderness over the whole forearm and elbow.
- Stretch test is positive (passive stretching of the fingers are painful)
- Neurovascular deficit: +/−
- Pulse: Feeble or absent

Investigation: X-ray of elbow and measurement of compartment pressure.

Treatment:
- Immediately exploration—fasciotomy and release of compartment
- Pressure and limb elevation

Q How will you investigate and treat a case of fracture supracondylar humerus?

Investigation:
- X-ray of elbow—anteroposterior and lateral view
- For vascular injury—angiography
- For nerve injury—nerve conduction velocity (NCV)

(Median/radial/ulnar—most common is median nerve)

Treatment:

Conservative: Closed reduction under general anesthesia and above elbow plaster of Paris (POP) back slab.

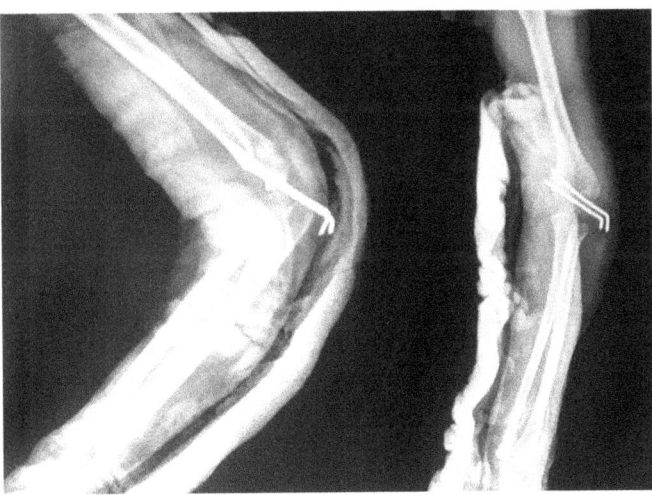

Operative: Classification of supracondylar fracture by Gartland's

Type I: Undisplaced—percutaneous pinning under image intensifier guidance

Type II: Minimally displaced—closed reduction and percutaneous pinning under image intensifier guidance

Type III: Complete displacement
- Closed reduction and percutaneous pinning by two parallel or
- Two cris-cross under image guide

Q What are the complication of fracture supracondylar humerus?

Complication:
- Immediate: Compartment syndrome with neurovascular deficit
- Delayed: Cubitus varus/valgus
    - Ulnar claw hand/pointing index (due to median nerve injury) or
    - Rarely wrist drop (due to radial nerve injury)
    - Joint stiffness at elbow joint
    - Depuytren's contracture

MEDIAL CONDYLE FRACTURE

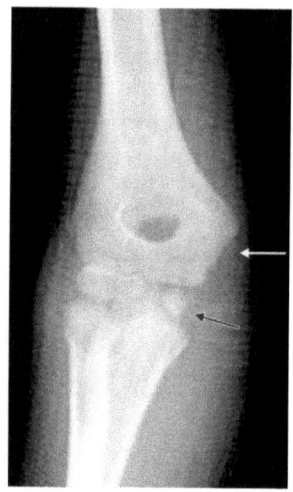

Q Write short notes on medial condyle fracture.

Mechanism of injury:
- Fall in outstretched hand and occurs in >5 years of age of child.
- In adult by road traffic accident (RTA) or fall.

Clinical features:
- Pain, swelling, restriction of elbow movements
- Tenderness over medial condyle

Investigation:
- X-ray of elbow (anteroposterior and lateral view)
- Nerve conduction velocity (NCV) study—to rule out ulnar nerve injury.

Treatment: Percutaneous pinning (two parallel K-wire) at medial condyle after closed reduction under image intensifier guidance.

LATERAL CONDYLE FRACTURE

Q Describe classification of lateral condyle of humerus fracture.

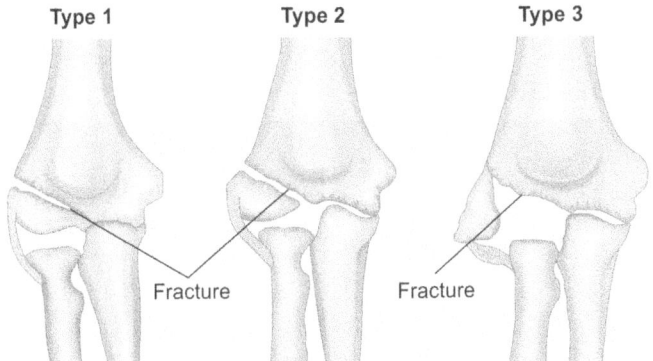

Classification of lateral condyle fracture

Type 1: Undisplaced fracture
Type 2: Minimally displaced fracture
Type 3: Displaced and rotated fracture

Q Describe mechanism of injury, clinical features, investigation and treatment of fracture lateral condyle of humerus.

Mechanism of injury:
- Fall in outstretched hand and occurs usually in 9-12 years of age of child.
- In adult by RTA or fall.

Clinical features:
- Pain, swelling, restriction of elbow movements.
- Tenderness over affected lateral condyle.

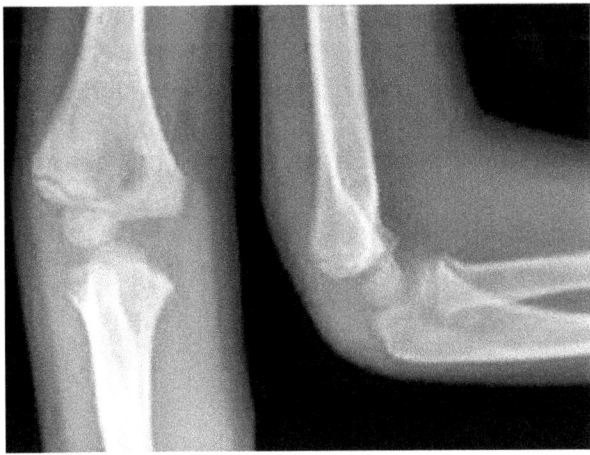

Investigation:
- X-ray of elbow (anteroposterior and lateral view)
- Nerve conduction velocity (NCV) study—to rule out radial or median nerve injury.

Treatment: Percutaneous pinning (two parallel K-wire) at lateral condyle after closed reduction under image intensifier guidance.

DISLOCATION OF ELBOW

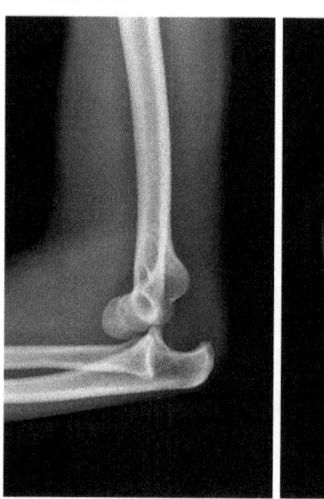
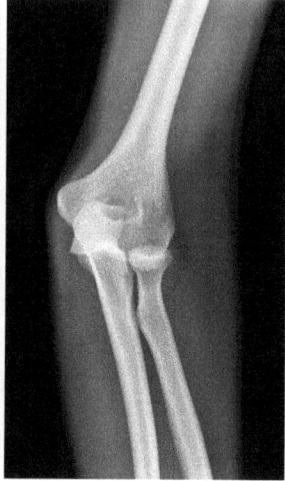

Q Write short notes on dislocation of elbow.

Mechanism of injury:
- Fall on outstretched hand with elbow in extension
- Cause posterior dislocation (90%)

Clinical features:
- Severe swelling, pain, deformity, tenderness +ve locally
- Abnormal bony landmarks
- Neurovascular injury ± (brachial artery, or median, ulnar or radial nerve may be injured.
- May be associated with fracture olecranon, fracture coronoid, fracture medial epicondyle.

Investigation: X-ray, color Doppler, angiography if vascular injury suspected.

Treatment:
- Urgent closed reduction under anesthesia and (above elbow) plaster of Paris (POP slab for 4–6 weeks.
- If any associated displaced fracture—open reduction and internal fixation (OR + IF) of that fracture.

Q Write complication of dislocation elbow.

Complication:
- Early:
  - Vascular (brachial artery) injury
  - Nerve (median/ulnar nerve) injury with associated fracture

- Late:
  - Myositis ossificans
  - Unreduced dislocation
  - Joint stiffness
  - Recurrent dislocation

RADIAL HEAD FRACTURE

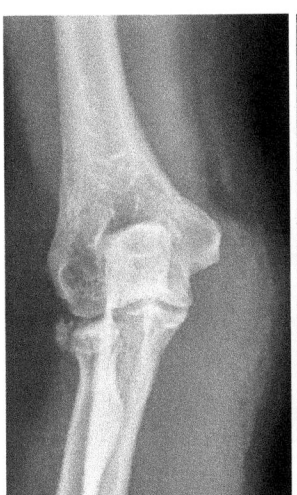 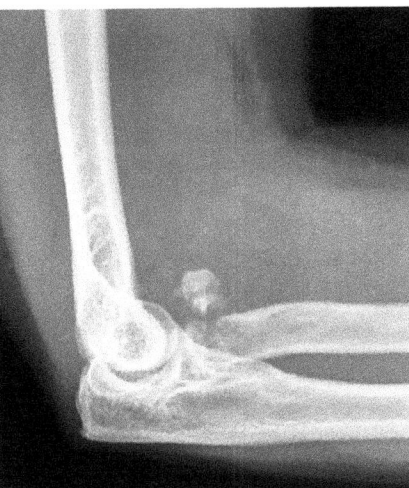

Q How to manage a case of fracture radial head?

Mechanism of injury:
- Fall in outstretched hand and occurs in 6–9 years of age (usually) of child.
- In adult by RTA or fall.

Clinical features:
- Pain, swelling, restriction of elbow movements
- Tenderness over affected radial head.

Investigation:
- X-ray of elbow (anteroposterior and lateral view)
- NCV study—to rule out radial or median nerve injury.

Treatment:
- If undisplaced fracture—arm support and gradual exercise, if no pain or swelling.
- If severe pain or swelling—then only above elbow POP slab is sufficient.
- If minimally displaced—percutaneous pinning after closed reduction under image intensifier guidance.
- If comminuted fracture—excision of small fragments
- In case large fragments—headless screws/Herbert's screw after open reduction, under image guidance.

FRACTURE OLECRANON

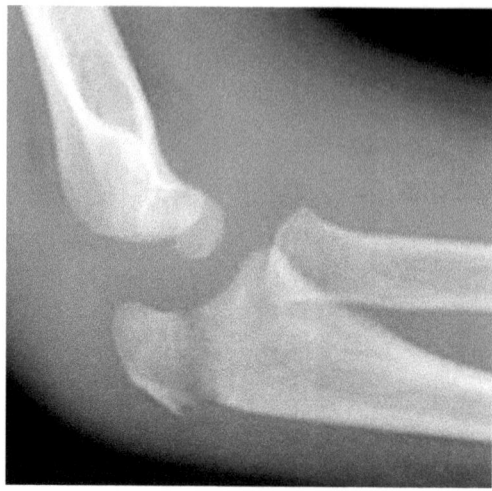

Q Write short notes on fracture olecranon.

Mechanism of injury
- Fall in outstretched hand and occurs in 6–10 years of age of child.
- In adult by RTA or fall.

Clinical features:
- Pain, swelling, restriction of elbow movements
- Tenderness over affected olecranon

Investigation:
- X-ray of elbow (anteroposterior and lateral view)
- NCV study—to rule out ulnar nerve injury

Treatment:
- If undisplaced fracture—only above elbow POP slab is sufficient.
- If minimally displaced—open reduction and internal fixation (ORIF) by tension band wiring (TBW—principle is conversion of tensile force to compressive force).

INTERCONDYLAR FRACTURE

Q Write short notes on intercondylar fracture of humerus.

Mechanism of injury: Commonly in adults followed by high velocity trauma.

Clinical features:
- Pain, swelling, restriction of elbow movements
- Tenderness over whole elbow

Investigation:
- X-ray of elbow (anteroposterior and lateral view)

- NCV study—to rule out any nerve injury
- Angiography—to rule out brachial artery injury.

Treatment: Open reduction and internal fixation (ORIF) by reconstruction plate.

CUBITUS VARUS AND VALGUS

Q Write short notes on cubitus varus/cubitus valgus.

Carrying angle of elbow is normally 5–10° (male) or 10–15° (female).

Etiology of varus:
- Supracondylar fracture—malunion
- Medial condyle fracture—malunion or nonunion.

Etiology of valgus:
- Lateral condyle fracture—malunion or nonunion
- Supracondylar fracture—malunion

Symptom:
- History of trauma followed by treatment.
- Complain of swelling and deformity on medial aspect (in case of varus).
- Complain of swelling and deformity on lateral aspect (in case of valgus).

Signs:
- Thickening of both supracondylar ridges in case of mal-united supracondylar fracture.
- Gunstock deformity (valgus)
- Three bonny point (lateral epicondyle, medial epicondyle, and olecranon) relationship is maintained (usually forms isosceles triangle).
- No restriction of movement (90% cases) in malunited supracondylar fracture.
- Restriction of movement in some cases due to fibrosis.

But if due to lateral or medial condylar fracture: Restriction of movements of elbow is present.

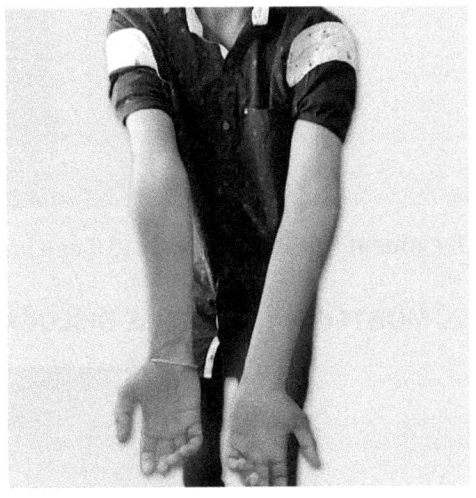

Cubitus Varus Lt elbow

Investigation: X-ray of both elbow (anteroposterior and lateral view)—draw carrying angle.

Treatment: Operative and plan is to

Get back the original carrying angle by corrective osteotomy
↓
Modified French osteotomy
Or
Dunn's osteotomy

FRACTURE BOTH BONE FOREARM

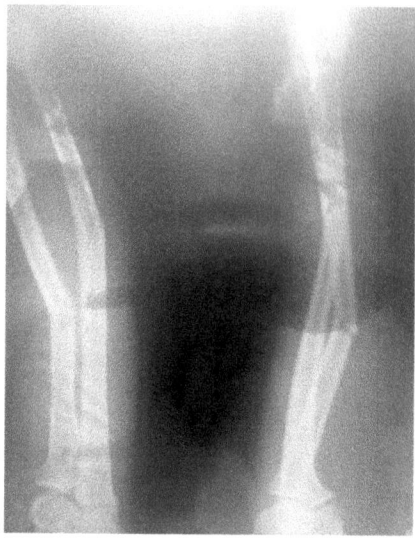

Treatment: ORIF with LCDCP (3.5 mm narrow) with cortical screw.

MONTEGGIA FRACTURE DISLOCATION

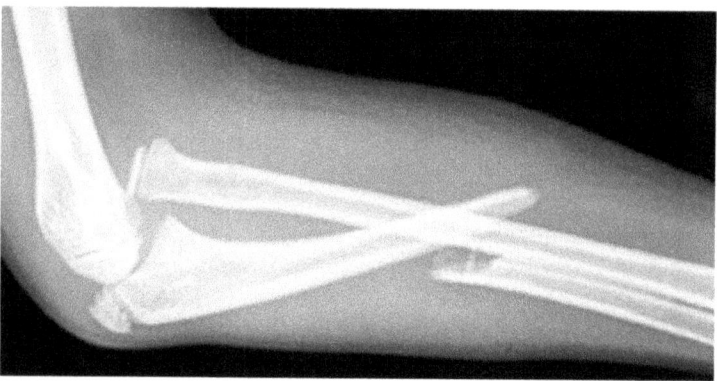

Q Write short notes on Monteggia fracture dislocation.

Fracture of proximal ulnar shaft with dislocation of head of radius.

Clinical features:
- Pain, swelling of proximal 1/3rd of forearm
- Restricted elbow

Treatment: Open reduction + internal fixation (ORIF) by plate (DCP/LCDCP) and with a K-wire through radiocapital joint.

GALEAZZI FRACTURE DISLOCATION

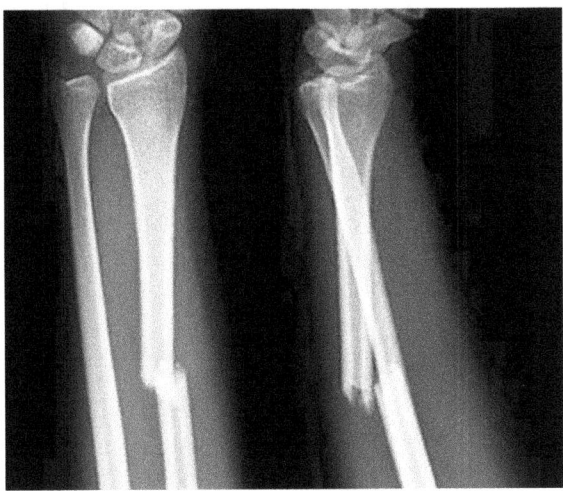

Q Write short notes on Galeazzi fracture dislocation.

Fracture of distal radius along with dislocation of inferior radioulnar joint.

Clinical features:
- Pain, swelling of wrist, i.e., distal forearm
- Restricted wrist movement

Investigation: X-ray—fracture with dislocation confirmed.

Treatment: OR + IF with plate (DCP/LCDCP) with a K-wire through inferior radioulnar joint after reduction.

CHAPTER 17: Fractures Around Wrist

COLLES FRACTURE

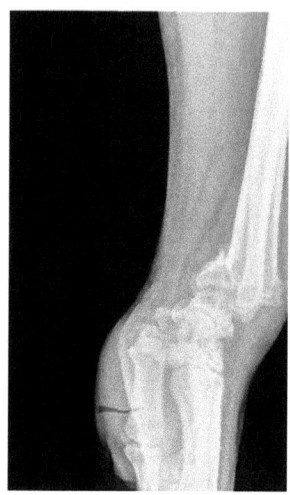

Q Write short notes on Colles' fracture.

Fracture or distal radius (extra-articular), occur usually >60 years age.

Clinical features: Pain, swelling, at wrist with restriction of movement and deformity (dinner-fork).

Investigation: X-ray—fracture at distal radius (no other fracture) within 2 cm from radial styloid.

Treatment:
- Closed reduction + plaster of Paris (POP) cast (below elbow)
- Closed reduction + percutaneous pin
- Closed reduction + external fixation by ligamentotaxis

Q What are the complication of Colles' fracture?

Complication:
- Wrist stiffness
- Sudeck's atrophy: It is a kind of reflex sympathetic dystrophy where swelling, tenderness of small joints of fingers leads to—stiff fingers
- X-ray shows osteoporosis and bone scan shows increase uptake
- Osteoporosis
- Secondary osteoarthritis (OA)

FRACTURE METACARPALS/FRACTURE PHALANGES

Q Write short notes on fracture metacarpals/fracture phalanges.

Clinical features: Pain, swelling, deformity, local tenderness at fracture side of metacarpals/phalanges.

Investigation: X-ray of hand (anteroposterior and lateral view)

Treatment:
- Undisplaced fracture—ball bandage
- Displaced fracture—closed reduction + internal fixation (CR+IF/open reduction + internal fixation (OR+IF) with K-wire under image guidance.

SCAPHOID FRACTURE

Q Write short notes on fracture scaphoid.

Mechanism of injury: Fall on dorsiflexed hand, mostly stable fracture.

Clinical features:
- Pain, swelling, at wrist
- Tenderness positive at anatomical snuff box—diagnostic sign
- Range of movements (ROM) of wrist—restricted.

Investigation:

X-ray wrist:
- Anteroposterior view
- Lateral view
- Oblique view
- Scaphoid view

Treatment:
- Undisplaced fracture: By scaphoid cast in glass holding position for 4 weeks.
- Displaced fracture: OR+IF with headless screw under imager guidance.

Complication:
- Avascular necrosis (AVN)
- Non-union
- Secondary osteoarthritis of wrist

CHAPTER 18

Spinal Disorders

SLIPPED DISK

Q Write short notes on slipped disc.

Etiopathogenesis: It may be precipitated by local strain of sudden injury prolapsed material press on dura mater—causing referred pain and paresthesia—sometime weakness of limb muscles.

Clinical features:
- In cervical disk prolapse—pain and stiffness of neck.
- In lumbar disk—backache, sciatica pain, cauda equina compression may cause urinary retention:
  - Tenderness in midline of low back
  - Straight le raise (SLR)—restricted
  - Paresthesia, weakness of limb muscle in advanced stage.

Investigation:
- X-ray of local spine (anteroposterior and lateral view)—shows paravertebral spasm and straightening of spine.
- MRI of local spine—canal diameter can be measured and cord compression can be diagnosed.

Treatment:
- Bed rest, nonsteroidal anti-inflammatory drugs (NSAIDs), muscle relaxant.
- Supportive brace
- Epidural injection of methyl prednisolone and local anesthetic.
- Operative:
  - Parital laminectomy
  - Laminotomy + dissectomy
  - Microdissectomy

KYPHOSCOLIOSIS

Q Write short notes on kyphoscoliosis.

It is a combine spinal disorder with kyphosis and scoliosis.

Types:
1. Congenital
2. Secondary

Spinal Disorders

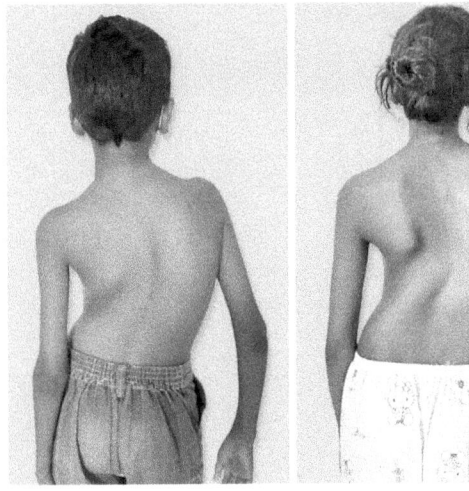

Scoliosis at child   Scoliosis at adult

- Adolescent
- Postural
- Osteoporosis
- Tuberculosis

Clinical features:
- Patient complaining of pain swelling at back with deformity
- Gibbus mostly present
- Hypoesthesia/numbness due to cord compression/damage.
- Coin test positive in tuberculosis (TB) spine (bends his hip, knee rather back).

Investigation: X-ray whole spine
- Anteroposterior (AP)
- Lateral

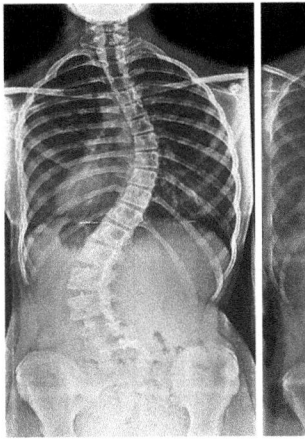 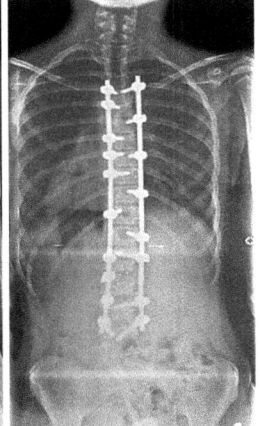

Before surgery   After surgery with pedicle screw with rod fixation

Determination of Cobb's angle for prognosis:
- Blood: Routine examination
- Mantoux test (+ve) in TB, mostly
- MRI of dorsolateral (DL) spine
- Needle biopsy if secondary

Treatment: Conservative treatment by:
- Milwaukee brace
- Boston brace

Operative: Posterior column stabilization by:
- Pedicle screw fixation
- Harrington instrumentation
- Sub-laminar wiring

CERVICAL SPONDYLOSIS

Q Write short notes on cervical spondylosis.

Clinical features: Most common disorder of cervical spine:
- Patients of >40 years cause of neck pain with paresthesia or weakness of upper limb.
- Tenderness in posterior neck muscles with painful and limited neck movements.
- Deep reflexes may be depressed in case of numbness of limb.

Investigation:
- X-ray—narrowing of disk space with osteophyte at the margin of disk.
- MRI—to know the exact picture of spinal canal.

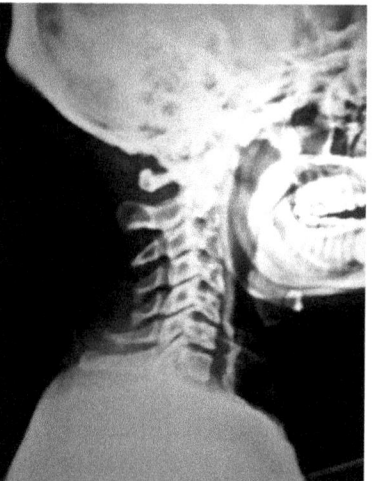

Treatment:
- Heat
- Cervical collar
- NSAIDs with muscle relaxant
- Physiotherapy—gentle manipulation and intermittent traction

SPONDYLOLISTHESIS

Q Describe spondylolisthesis.

Defination: Forward shift of spine, commonly occurs at L5-S1 or L4-L5

Types:
1. Lytic (50%)
2. Degenerative (25%)

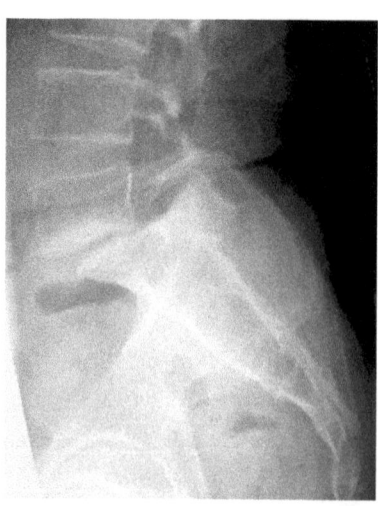

3. Dysplastic
4. Post-traumatic

Pathology: In lytic type:
- Pars intra-articularis is in two pieces and the gap is occupied by fibrous tissue.
- Behind the gap:
  - Spinous process
  - Laminae and inferior articular facet remain as separate fragment.
- With stress—vertebral body and superior facets in front of gap may subluxate or dislocate forwards—carrying vertebral column with it and put pressure on dura/cauda equine.

Clinical features:
- Usually patients of >50 years cause of backache, with sciatica or pseudoclaudication due to spinal stenosis.
- On examination—flattening of buttock, with prominent transverse loin creases, scoliosis +/-, Hamstring tightness.

Investigation:
- X-ray—forward shift of upper part of spinal column
- MRI—to rule out spinal cord compression

Treatment:
- Physiotherapy, lumbosacral (LS) corset, activity modification, NSAIDs, with muscle relaxants, facet joint injections.
- Operative: If slip >50%—then decompression and spinal stabilization by pedicle screw fixation.

CHAPTER 19

Short Notes

BRODIE'S ABSCESS

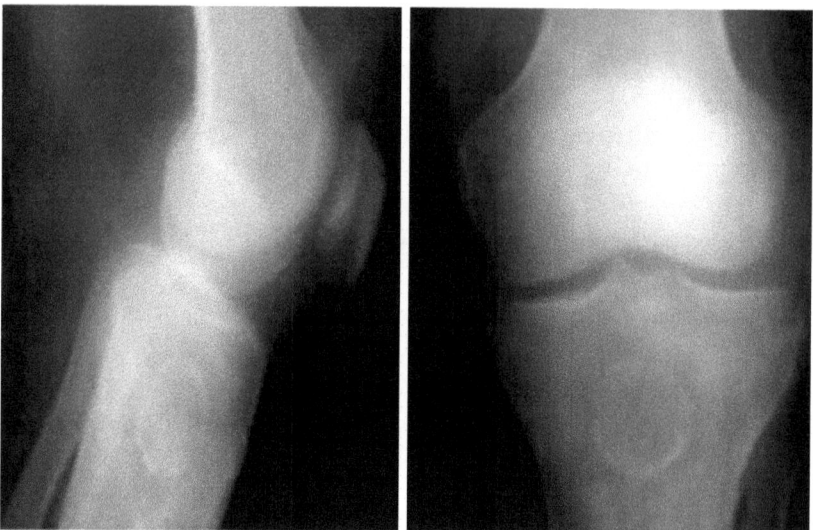

It is a type of chronic osteomyelitis.

Clinical features:

Symptoms: Fever and pain, swelling, redness locally at limb.

Signs:
- Tenderness (local), pyrexia, flares, or with discharging sinus
- Folded or puckered skin with excoriation.

Investigation: X-ray
- Area of osteolysis, surrounded by sclerotic bone with or without sequestrum
- Area of osteoporosis
- Periosteal thickening

Treatment:
- Corticotomy + drainage of pus
- Fill the cavity with antibiotic impregnated bone graft
- Immobilization for 1 month
- With intravenous antibiotics

MADE LUNG'S DEFORMITY

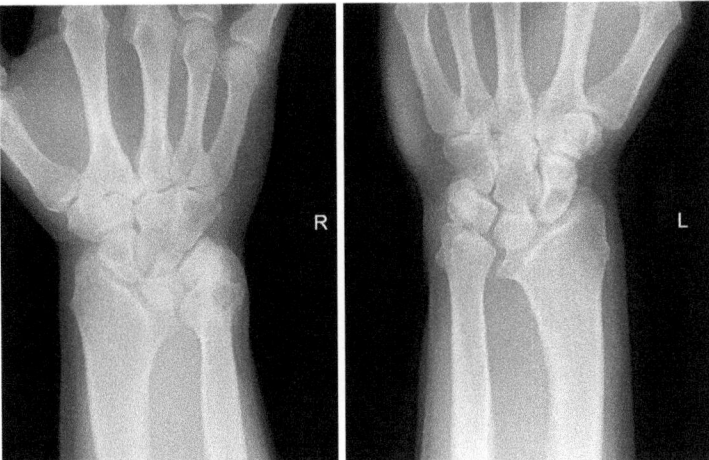

In this deformity—lower radius curves forwards, carrying with it corpus and hand, leaving lower ulna in its position.

Etiology: Mostly
- Congenital (as a part of general dysplasia)
- May be post-traumatic

Clinical features:
- The deformity rarely seen before 10 years, though present since birth.
- Presented with swelling (painless usually)
- Function of wrist is usually excellent.

Investigation:
- X-ray of wrist—anteroposterior (AP)/lateral view
- Nerve conduction velocity (NCV) study of affected limb.

Treatment:
- Darrach's procedure—excision of lower end of ulna.
- Sometimes corrective osteotomy of radius is required.

RADIAL CLUB HAND

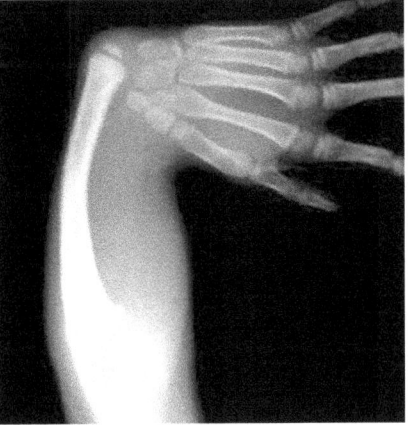

Clinical features:
- Absent of whole part of radius, thumb and sometimes first 2 rays of hand.
- May occur a part of generalized dysplasia.
- Congenital deformity
- Deformity of wrist and hand without any pain.

Investigation: X-ray of wrist.

Treatment:
- In neonate—manipulation and splintage
- In child (operative)—centralization of carpus over ulna (before 3 years)

ULNAR CLUB HAND

Due to complete or partial absence of ulna.

Clinical features:
- Deformity at ulnar side of forearm
- Ulnar ray may be missing
- Radial head may dislocate

Treatment:
- Stretching and splintage
- In severe deformity—excision of ulnar anlage and osteotomy of radius.

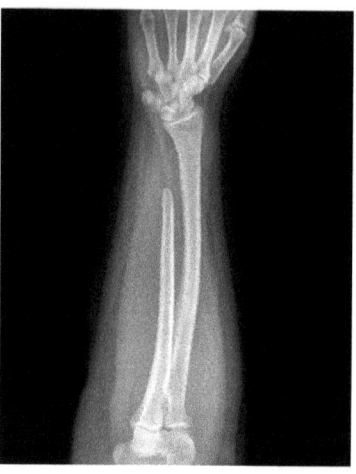

BONE TUMORS OF CARTILAGE ORIGIN

Q Write short notes of bone tumors of cartilage origin.
- Chondroma
- Periosteal chondroma
- Osteochondroma
- Chondromyxoid fibroma
- Chondroblastoma
- Chondrosarcoma (cartilage capped exostosis)

CARPAL TUNNEL SYNDROME

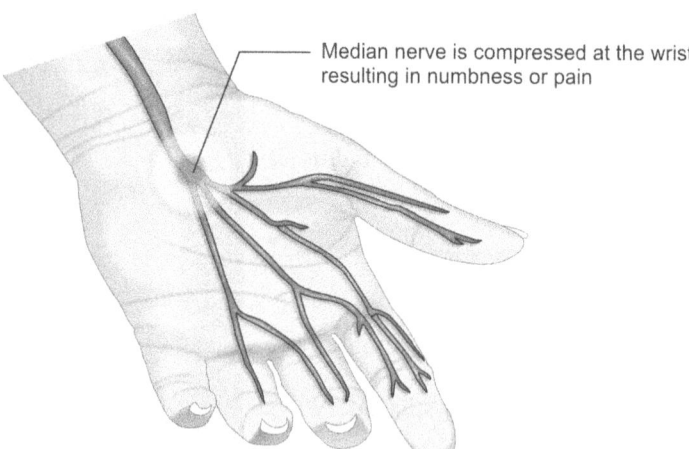

Median nerve is compressed at the wrist, resulting in numbness or pain

Commonly affected in female (menopause), in pregnancy, in myxoedema.

Clinical features:

Symptoms:
- Complaining of pain, swelling at wrist and fingers.
- Tingling, numbness of fingers
- Patient awake in midnight due to pain.

Signs:
- Tenderness at carpal tunnel (palmar aspect)
- Wasting of thenar muscle
- Forced palmar flexion—induce pain or tingling
- Map test: Asking the patient to mark affected areas, which
  ↓
  Corresponds distribution of median nerve

Investigation:
- X-ray cervical spine (AP/lateral view)—cervical spondylosis
- Nerve conduction velocity study.

Treatment: Conservative wrist splintage at night.

Operative: Division of carpal tunnel and decompression of median nerve.

DE QUERVAIN'S DISEASE

Etiology: Painful thickening of tendon sheath containing extensor policis bravis and abductor policis longus, at distal radius.

Clinical features: Female (40–50 years), complaining of—pain at wrist (radial side)
- Difficulties in wringing of clothes
- Swelling over distal radius
- Palpable thick tendon sheath
- Tenderness at tip of radial styloid
- Finkelstein's sign—+ve (abduction of thumb against resistant)

Investigation: X-ray of wrist—osteoarthritis or old fractures of scaphoid may be present.

Treatment:

Conservative:
- Local infiltration of corticosteroid at affected tendon sheath.
- Plaster splintage of wrist.

Operative: In resistant cases—slitting of thick tendon sheath.

ANKYLOSIS

Types:
1. Bony
2. Fibrous

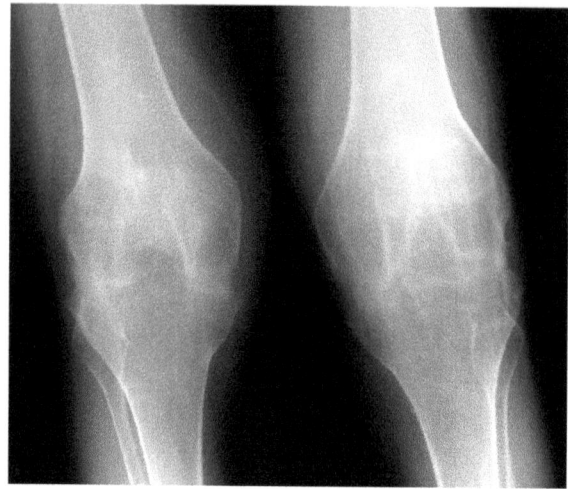

Etiology:
- Fracture followed by trauma—bony
- Infection—fibrous
- Non-union in fracture—fibrous

Clinical features:
- *Bony ankylosis*
  - Painless
  - Swelling (severe)
  - Gross restriction of movement of nearby joint or stiff joint.
- *Fibrous ankylosis*
  - Pain severe
  - Swelling present
  - Tenderness present
  - Jog of movement is possible

Investigation:
- X-ray of affected joint (AP/lateral)
- Blood for routine examination (RE), erythrocyte sedimentation rate (ESR), C-reactive protein (CRP)
- Tissue culture

Treatment:
- If bony ankylosis—reconstruction of joint (hip/knee) by total hip replacement (THR) and total knee replacement (TKR)
- If fibrous ankylosis—debridement and antibiotic/physiotherapy.

FROZEN SHOULDER

Etiology:
- Idiopathic
- Minor trauma may be a precipitating factor.

Clinical features:
- Age: 40–60 years usually
- Pain and stiffness at shoulder
- Tenderness, restricted movement—abduction and internal rotation.

Investigation:
- X-ray shoulder (AP/lateral)
- MRI shoulder
- Arthography shows contracted joint

Treatment:
- **U**sually resolves spontaneously after 18 months
- NSAIDs and "pendulum" exercise
- Injection of corticosteroid and ultrasonic therapy (UST)

If no relief:
- Manipulation under anesthesia
- Arthroscopy

BONE GRAFT

Indication:
- Non-union
- To fill up tumor cavity
- To fill up dead space in chronic osteomyelitis after saucerization

Types:
1. According to vascularity
   - Vascularized
   - Avascular
2. According to donor
   - Autogenous—from same patient
   - Allogenous—from different patient
   - Xenograft—from same species
3. According to osteogenic tissue
   - Cortical
   - Cancellous
   - Corticocancellous

Sites for autogenous graft:
- Iliac crest
- Tibia
- Olecranon
- Ribs

RUPTURED TENDO-ACHILLES

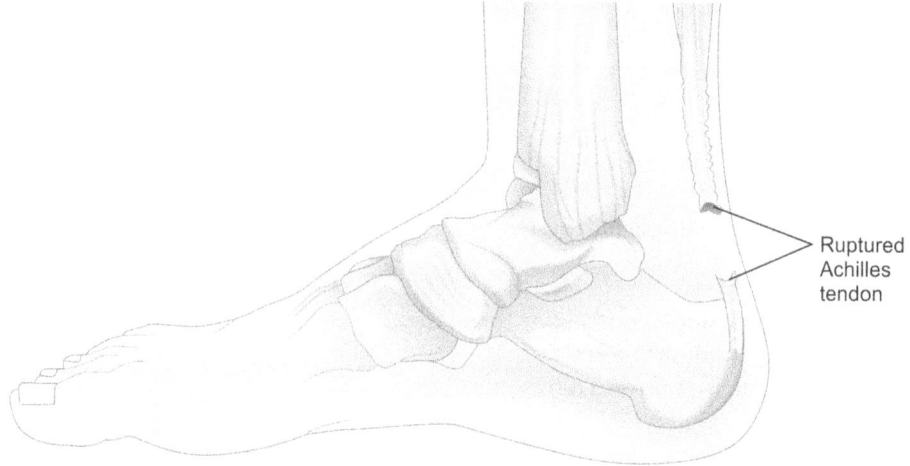
Ruptured Achilles tendon

Occur due to degeneration >40 years age.

Mechanism of injury (tendo-Achilles):
- It is the mulsculotendinous part of gastrosoleus muscle and inserted at calcaneal tuberosity.
- During running/jumping
- Calf muscle contracts
- Body weight resists that
- Tendon ruptures

Clinical features:
- Pain, swelling at heel and gap felt 5 cm above tendon insertion
- Weak plantar flexion
- Simond test—positive

Investigation: X-ray, USG of heel.

Treatment: Operative (by small transverse incision) repair + equinus plaster × 8 weeks.

MALLET FINGER

Etiopathogenesis:
- Injury to extensor tendon of distal phalanx due to direct trauma.
- Avulsion fracture of distal phalanx may occur.

Clinical features:
- Pain, swelling at distal interphalangeal joint (DIP)
- DIP joint is flexed and tender
- Patient cannot do active extention but passive is possible
- Proximal interphalangeal joint (PIP) is extended or may be hyperextended

Investigation:
- X-ray of local part—anteroposterior (AP) and lateral
- USG of local part

Treatment:
- Splintage in extension by Mallet finger splint in acute case.
- For old case—excision of ellipse of skin extensor tendon over terminal knuckle—defect is tightly sutures and hold the joint by K-wire.

TRIGGER FINGER

Etiopathogenesis:
- Flexor tendon may be trapped at its sheath entrance
- Forceful extension is possible by a snap (triggering)
- Usually cause is thickening of fibrous tendon sheath due to trauma/local unaccustomed activity.

Clinical features:
- Patient notices clicking of the finger as he bends it
- Affected finger remain bend
- Tender nodule positive

Treatment:
- Local infiltration of methyl prednisolone at tendon sheath entrance.
- If refractory (operative)—transverse incision at distal palmar crease.

CODMANN'S TRIANGLE

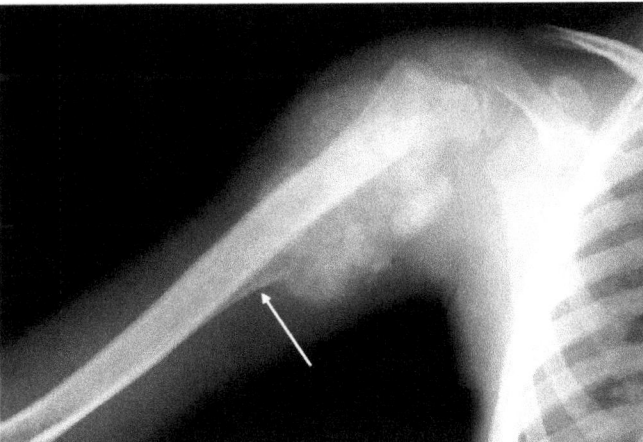

It is radiological feature in osteosarcoma (typical) and can be seen in Ewing's tumor or chronic osteomyelitis.

Etiopathogenesis:
- Where the tumor emerges from cortex
- Reactive now bone forms at the angles of periosteal elevation like triangle.

Investigation: X-ray of osteosarcoma.

Treatment:
- Confirmation of tumor by incisional biopsy
- Operative and radiotherapy/chemotherapy.

BONE SCAN

Mainly technetium labeled hydroxymethylene diphosphonate (^{99m}TC HDP) is injected intravenous (IV) route and its activity recorded in two stages.

1. Blood pool phase (immediate after injection): Increased uptake in acute or chronic synovitis and decreased uptake in local vascular insufficiency.
2. Bone phase (3 hours after injection): Increased uptake in fractures, infection, local tumor, healing after necrosis and decreased uptake in head of femur after fracture neck of femur (NOF).

CLINICAL APPLICATION

- Stress fracture, bone abscess, osteoid osteoma, Perthes disease, avascular necrosis (AVN), infection, and early diagnosis in metastasis.
- Other radionuclides used are ^{99m}TC-Sc, ^{67}Ga, ^{111}In.

HOUSEMAID'S KNEE

Uninfected prepatellar bursitis in a normal knee joint.

Clinical features:
- Fluctuant, circumscribed
- Swelling in front of patella

Treatment:
- Firm bandage, avoid, kneeling
- Nonsteroidal anti-inflammatory drugs (NSAIDs) if pain
- Aspiration occasionally
- Exicision in chronic case of lump

BAKER'S CYST

Popliteal cyst occurs due to synovial rupture in a diseased joint [may be osteoarthritis (OA)/rheumatoid arthritis (RA)].

Clinical fractures:
- Swelling
- Nontender lump at midline of popliteal fossae
- Fluctuation +ve bellow joint line

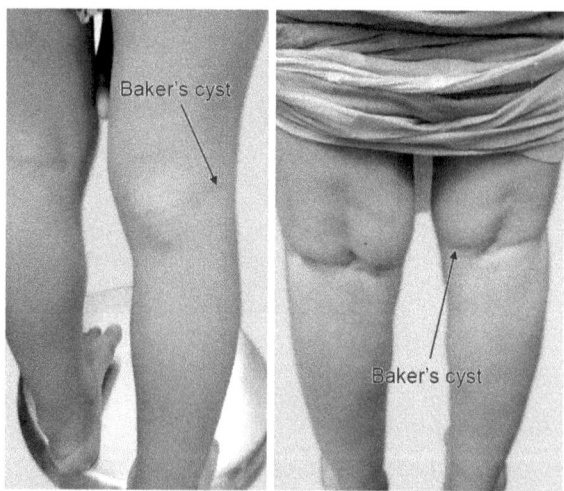

Treatment:
- Aspiration and local infiltration of methyl prednisolone
- Synovectomy in chronic case

ARTHROSCOPY

Use:
- Accuracy of diagnosis
- For taking decision, when to operate
- To record the progression of knee disorder
- To perform operative procedure [anterior cruciate ligament (ACL)/posterior cruciate ligament (PCL) reconstruction]

Technique:
- Regional anesthesia + tourniquet
- Saline injected
- Trocar and cannula introduced in a mini-incision
- Penetration of synovium
- All knee compartments are visible by light source and camera

Surgery done:
- Biopsy, partial menisectomy,
- Patellar shaving, loose body removal
- Synovectomy, ligaments replacement

Complication:
- Knee effusion
- Hemarthrosis
- Infection (1–2%)

TARDY ULNAR NERVE PALSY/ULNAR CLAW HAND

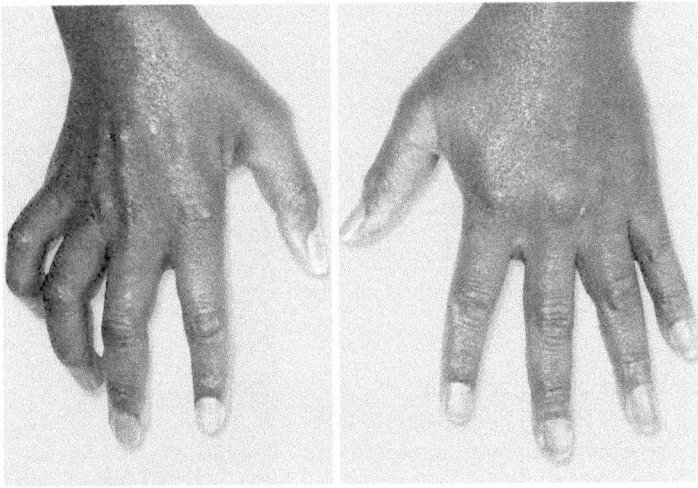

It is sequel of elbow disorders like OA elbow, cubitus valgus.

Clinical features:
- Numbness, weakness of hand
- Clawing
- Wasting interossei (mainly 1st)
- Tenderness positive over nerve in elbow

Investigation:
- Nerve conduction velocity (NCV) study
- Plain X-ray of elbow
- Magnetic resonance imaging (MRI)

Treatment: Decompression of ulnar nerve by dividing the root of ulnar tunnel in long incision, followed by (AE) POP slab for 3 weeks.

WRIST DROP

It is a sequel of radial nerve palsy.

Clinical features:
- Loss of flexion and active extension of wrist
- No local tenderness
- Skin of wrist is shiny, hair loss present
- Wasting of thenar, hypothenar muscles in chronic cases

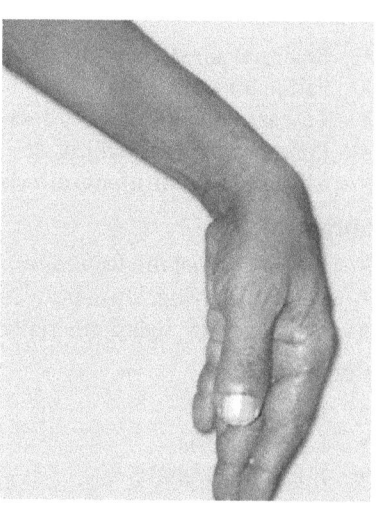

Investigation:
- NCV study
- Plain X-ray

Treatment:

Conservative:
- By dynamic cock-up splint
- Injection methylcobalamine, injection methylprednisolone

Operative: Tendon transfer.

MYOSITIS OSSIFICANS

Ossification of muscle tissue

Etiology: Following trauma /massage

Clinical features
- Patient develops a painful swelling at the proximity to joint.
- Tender swelling
- On palpation—firm to hard swelling
- Range of movement (ROM)—restricted initially
- Commonly on occur in elbow proximity in fracture around elbow.

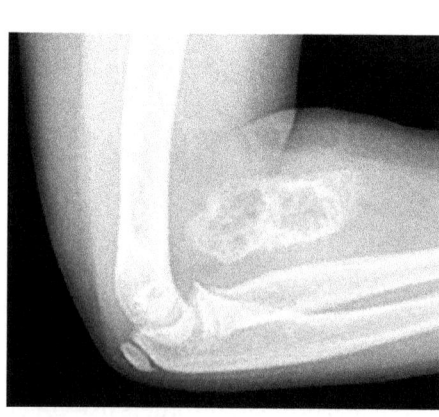

Investigation:
- X-ray of the affected part—showing new bone formation
- Fluffy density in soft tissue

Treatment:
- Rest
- Splintage
- No manipulation
- Nonsteroidal anti-inflammatory drugs (NSAIDs)

Classification:
1. Traumatica (most common)
2. Progressiva
3. Congenita

TENNIS ELBOW

Etiology: Repetitive strains at common tendon origin of wrist extensor.

Clinical features:
- Pain and swelling at lateral aspect of elbow
- Tenderness positive at lateral epicondyle

Pathology: Microscopic tearing of aponeurosis by local inflammation or vascular congestion or crystal deposition.

Investigation: X-ray of elbow—no abnormality detected (NAD)

Treatment:
- Rest/splintage
- NSAIDs
- Local injection of corticosteroids
- But if frequently recurs

GOLFER'S ELBOW

Etiology: Repetitive strains at common tendon origin of wrist flexor.

Clinical features:
- Pain and swelling at medial aspect of elbow
- Tenderness positive at medial epicondyle

Pathology: Microscopic tearing of aponeurosis by local inflammation or vascular congestion or crystal deposition.

Investigation: X-ray of elbow— No abnormality detected (NAD)

Treatment:
- Rest/splintage
- NSAIDs

- Local injection of corticosteroids
- But if frequently recurs

VOLKMANN'S ISCHEMIC CONTRACTURE

It is the ischemic contracture of the affected muscle following compartment syndrome or vascular injury.

Clinical features: Most common affected side—forearm and hand, leg and foot deformity due to contracture of forearm muscle stiffness

- Stiffness of fingers/wrist
- Numbness of fingers
- Wasting of forearm hand muscle
- Clawing of fingers (in severe case)

Investigation:

- X-ray of wrist forearm and hand—anteroposterior and lateral
- NCV study
- Electronystagmography (ENG) study

Treatment:

- Physiotherapy
- Operative:
  - MaxPage operation: Detachment of flexors at origin and along interosseous membrane
- Pedicle nerve graft may restore sensation
- Tendons transfer—can grasp (wrist extensors to finger and thumb flexors).

GANGLION

Etiology:

- Due to cystic degeneration of capsule or fibrous sheath
- The cyst having viscous fluid

Clinical features:

- Young adult, with a painless lump, in wrist (most common)
- Lump is cystic, well defined, nontender
- May be transilluminated
- May cause numbness (if nerve is close to it)

Treatment:

- Disappear spontaneously
- If any numbness still present—operative removal of ganglion

CHAPTER 20

Practical Examination (Orthopedics)

LONG CASES

1. **Hip case**
   - Nonunion fracture (NOF)
   - Chronic osteomyelitis in long bone
   - Perthes disease
   - Tuberculosis (TB) hip
   - Neglected dislocation of hip
   - Post-septic sequelae of hip
2. **Spine case:** TB spine or Koch's spine/or caries spine

HISTORY TAKING/WRITING: IN A LONG CASE OF HIP

Please keep in mind that history writing and its presentation like a story to examiner is an art.

1. **Patient's particular:** Name, age, sex, address, literacy level of patient—write separately but present in a single sentence.
2. **Chief complaints:** Patient may not tell but you should try to elicit about the followings:
   - Pain at hip with duration
   - Limping of limb with duration
   - Restriction of movement of hip
   - Shortening of affected limb
   - Swelling, if present
3. **History of present illness:** Patient was apparently all right before (say about the period of normal being or time of trauma):
   1st paragraph: Elaboration of all points of chief complaints with duration and chronological order, e.g.,
   - Pain—onset, site, character, radiation to knee or ankle, aggravating or relieving factor, with duration
   - Limping—progressive or nonprogressive with duration
   - Restriction of movement—in the form of difficulty in squatting, cross leg sitting on the floor, or stair climbing with duration,
   - Shortening—progressive or nonprogressive with duration
   - Swelling—progressive or nonprogressive

   2nd paragraph: Any history of evening rise of temperature, cough and cold, anorexia, weight loss (common in TB hip).

   3rd paragraph: Any history of night cry (common in TB hip) or history of morning stiffness (in rheumatoid arthritis, ankylosing spondylitis, gouty arthritis).

4th paragraph: Any drug history of prolonged drug intake (e.g., ATD, steroid, antiepileptics) and any family history of pulmonary tuberculosis.

5th paragraph: Personal history, e.g., sleep, appetite, menstrual history in female.

4. **General Survey:**
   - Consciousness, orientation
   - Build, height, weight, nutrition
   - Anemia, jaundice, cyanosis, clubbing
   - Pulse, blood pressure (BP), respiration, temperature

5. **Local examination of pathological hip:** I have examined the patient in standing, sitting and lying position, from front, side and back.
   a. **On inspection:**
      - Attitude of affected lower limb—flexed, abducted or adducted, or rotated externally/internally
      - Acromial and scapular angle at same level or high up in any side
      - Dorsal spine—any kyphosis or scoliosis
      - Lumbar spine—lumbar lordosis is exaggerated or not, if exaggerated, which is compensated by FFD of hip or fixed flexion deformity (concealed deformity)
      - Both anterior superior iliac spine (ASIS) and posterior superior iliac spine (PSIS)—at same level or not
      - Both greater trochanter (GT) at same level or migrated up or down
      - Patella or medial malleoli tip—same or shifted
      - Muscle wasting—search for quadricep's or Hamstring's wasting.
   b. **On palpation:** All bony points inspected are confirmed by palpation, we divide the hip in four quadrants:
      1. Medially—look for adductor spasm—present in TB hip or post-septic sequelae
      2. Anteriorly—temperature, tenderness at anterior hip point, vascular sign of Narath (-ve in presence of pulsation of femoral artery and +ve in absence or feeble pulse in neglected hip dislocation or post-septic sequelae), and inguinal or deep external iliac group of lymph node
      3. Laterally—surface, tenderness, widening and broadening, migration of greater trochanter of pathological side should assess, as compare to normal hip. Migration can be assessed by digital Bryant's triangle.
      4. Posteriorly—should see for any hard globular bony mass palpable in posterior hip joint, if mass present—that is probably dislocated femoral head.
   c. **Movement of affected hip:** 1st do squaring of pelvis, look for any fixed deformity:
      - Normal hip
        * Flexion—0 to 140 degree
        * Extension—0 to 15 degree
        * Abduction—0 to 45 degree
        * Adduction—0 to 40 degree
        * External rotation—0 to 50 degree
        * Internal rotation—0 to 40 degree
      - If fixed adduction deformity (measured by Kothari's angle) present—no abduction, scoliosis and apparent shortening of pathological limb.

- If fixed abduction deformity present—no adduction, scoliosis in opposite side and apparent lengthening of pathological limb.
d. **Measurement:**
   - Apparent length of limb—from xiphisternum to medial malleoli tip and compare with normal limb.
   - True length of limb—from ASIS to tip of medial malleoli and compare with normal limb.
e. **Special tests:**
   - Thomas test—to reveal fixed flexion deformity (FFD) of hip
   - Telescopic test—positive in fracture neck of femur (NOF)
   - Trendelenberg's test—positive in abductor weakness.
f. **Gait:** Antalgic (painful) or short limp (limp without pain) or Trendelenberg gait (Trendelenberg's test positive) usually present.
6. Examination of ipsilateral knee and ankle
7. Examination of contralateral hip, knee, and ankle
8. Spine examination
9. Provisional diagnosis
10. Differential diagnosis
11. Investigation
12. Summary of the long case in 5 or 6 line

NONUNION FRACTURE NECK OF FEMUR

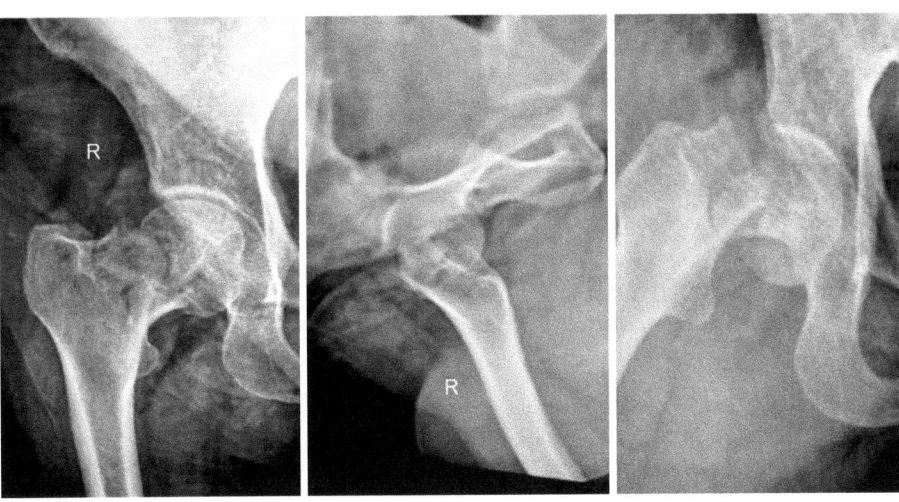

From history:
- History of trivial trauma long back—followed by pain, difficulty in walking with limping.
- No history of fever, cough, cold with weight loss.

General survey:
- Patient is conscious, oriented
- Pallor ±

Clinical examination of affected hip:

Inspection:
- Attitude—affected limb is externally rotated
- Shortening may be visible
- Wasting of glutei, quadriceps, Hamstrings of affected limb.

Palpation:
- Local tenderness ±
- Widening, broadening of greater trochanter (GT)
- Digital Bryant's triangle—showed proximal migration of affected GT
- No hard globular bony mass palpable at posterior aspect of hip

Range of movement:
- Fixed flexion deformity (FFD) ±—compensated by exaggerated lumbar lordosis confirmed by Thomas test
- Flexion—usually restricted terminally due to fibrosis or muscle contracture
- Fixed abduction deformity ±
- Fixed external rotation deformity positive in long standing case

Measurement:
- Apparent shortening—in fixed adduction deformity
- Apparent lengthening—in fixed abduction deformity
- True shortening : +ve

Special test:
- Thomas test: +ve if FFD
- Telescopic test: +ve
- Trendelenberg test: +ve [criteria—patient has to stand on affected hip for 30 seconds at least) and pathological side posterior superior iliac spine (PSIS) will go upwards, instead drooping downwards]

Provisional diagnosis: Nonunion fracture NOF.

Differential diagnosis:
- Nonunion fracture trochanter
- Slipped capital femoral epiphysis in child

Investigation:
- X-ray of pelvis of both hip (anteroposterior)
- X-ray affected hip with thigh (lateral)
- MRI of hip to see any avascular necrosis (AVN) of femur head and acetabulum.

Summary:

TUBERCULOSIS OF HIP

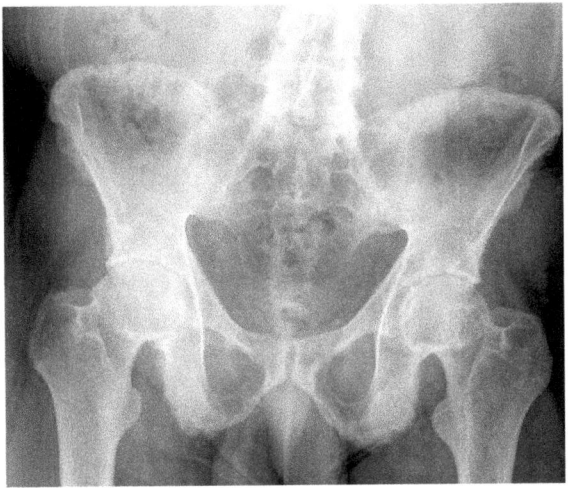

From history:
- History of severe pain, swelling, deformity of affected hip at least 2-3 month duration
- History of restricted movement of hip
- History of cough, cold, evening rise of temperature (low grade) and weight loss
- Family history of TB ±
- Any prolonged drug intake like ATD or steroid, previously for pulmonary Koch's

General survey:
- Patient is conscious oriented
- Build, height—average
- Nutrition—may be below average
- Pallor: ++

Clinical examination:

Inspection:
- Attitude—is flexed, adducted (usually) of affected limb
- Muscle wasting—of glutei, quadriceps, Hamstring muscles
- Visible shortening ± of the limb

Palpation:
- Adductor spasm +ve
- Severe tenderness +ve at anterior hip point
- Tenderness ++ over greater trochanter also
- Palpable and significant inguinal and external iliac group of lymph nodes

Movements of affected hip:
- Restricted in all direction with FFD or
- Fixed abduction deformity (early stage) or
- Fixed adduction deformity (late stage) and fixed rotational deformity.

If FFD present—compensatory exaggerated lumbar lordosis also there.

If fixed adduction deformity—apparent shortening.

If fixed abduction deformity—apparent lengthening present.

Measurement: Apparent shortening or lengthening according to fixed adduction or abduction deformity.

Provisional diagnosis: Tuberculosis of hip.

Differential diagnosis:
- Perthes disease
- Transient synovitis of hip
- Monoarticular RA (rheumatoid arthritis only one joint affected)

Investigation:
- X-ray pelvis and both hip (anteroposterior)
- X-ray of affected hip, i.e., thigh (lateral)
- MRI of affected hip
- Blood for RE, erythrocyte sedimentation rate (ESR), C-reactive protein (CRP), rheumatoid arthritis (RA) factor, asitis anti-cyclic citrullinated peptide (anti-CCP)
- Polymerase chain reaction (PCR) for TB

Summary:

NEGLECTED DISLOCATION HIP

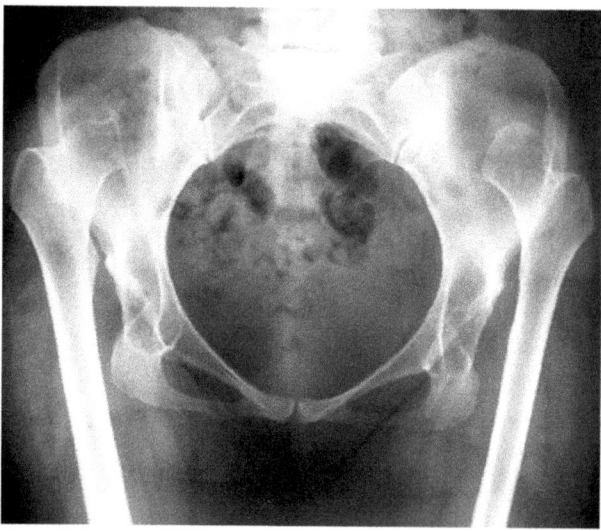

From history: History of severe trauma to hip long back, and not treated properly.
- Complain of pain, swelling, gross restriction of movement
- Shortening +ve
- No history of fever, cold, anorexia

Clinical examination:

Inspection:
- In posterior dislocation—attitude of limb is flexed, adducted, internally rotated
- Visible shortening
- Muscle wasting in neglected case

Palpation:
- Tenderness +ve at posterior hip joint line
- Vascular sign of Narath is +ve
- Hard globular bony mass palpable at posterior hip joint line of affected hip—most probably it is dislocated femoral head.

Range of movements: Grossly restricted all directions.

Measurement: True shortening positive.

Provisional diagnosis: Neglected dislocation of hip.

Differential diagnosis: Post-septic sequelae of hip.

Investigation: Same like fracture neck of femur (NOF)

Summary:

POST-SEPTIC SEQUELAE—USUALLY OCCURS IN CHILD

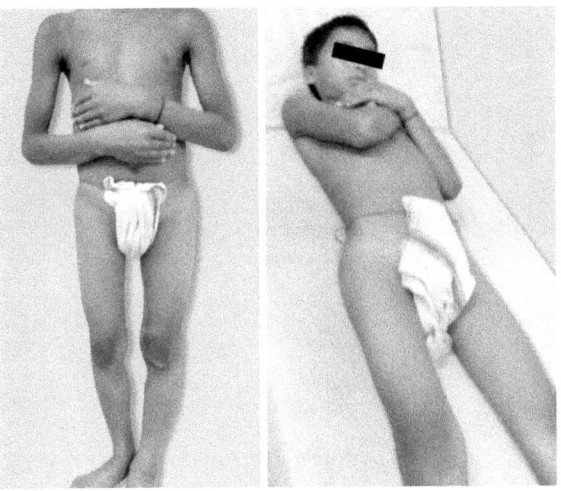

From history:
- History of septicemia, or prolonged high-grade fever
- Followed by weakness lower limb, i.e., affected side
- Pain, swelling, gross restriction of movement

Inspection:
- Attitude—Limb may externally rotated, or flexed
- Muscle wasting ±ve
- Adduction spasm ±ve

Palpation:
- Tenderness ± anterior joint line of hip
- Vascular sign of Narath ±ve
- Widening, broadening of affected greater trochanter, may be dislocated
- Palpable inguinal lymph nodes

Movements:
- Restricted in all direction, i.e., FFD, fixed abduction or adduction deformity.
- Fixed rotation deformity ±, according to involvement of group of muscles.

Measurement: True shortening ±ve

Special tests: Telescopic test +ve, if femoral head is completely absorbed by disease process.

Provisional diagnosis: A sequelae of septic arthritis of hip.

Differential diagnosis:
- Slipped capital femoral epiphysis
- Transient synovitis of hip

Investigation:
- X-ray
- MRI—to see epiphyseal or physeal part of femoral head
- Blood—R/E, ESR, CRP, PCR of TB

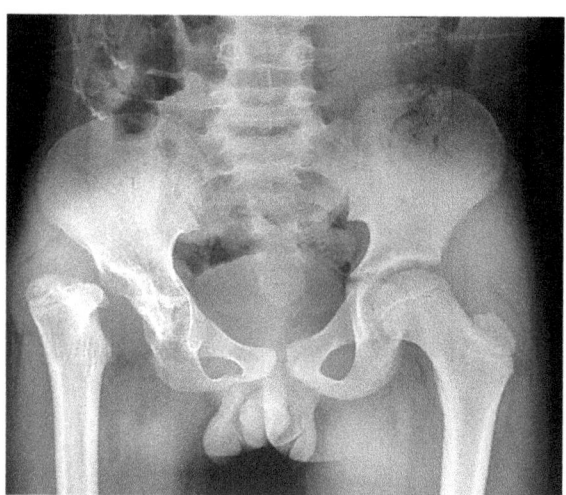

Summary:

CHRONIC OSTEOMYELITIS

From history:
- History of high-grade fever, septicemia, in near past or any surgery to bone
- Pain, swelling affected area
- History of discharging sinus

Practical Examination (Orthopedics) 113

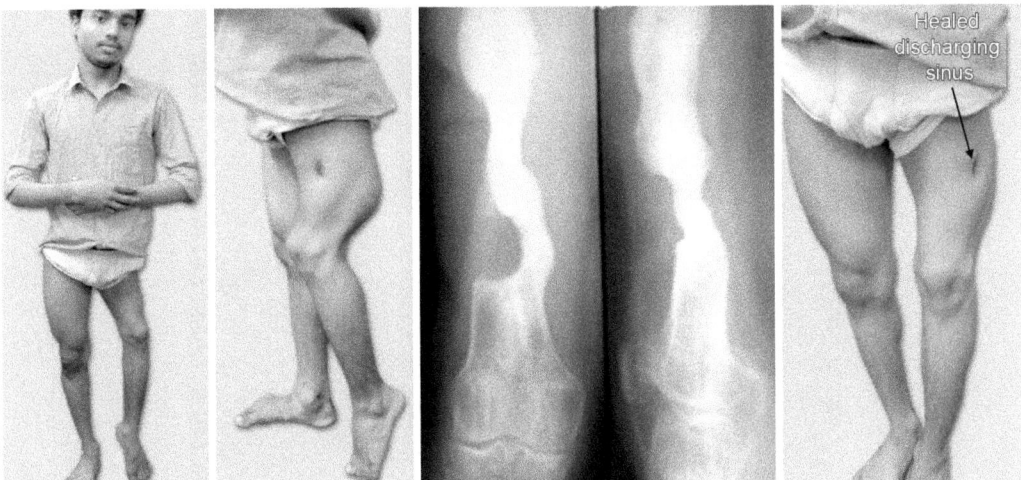

General survey: Pallor ++

Clinical examination:

Inspection:
- Any discharging sinus with inverted or everted margin, with skin fixity to underlying bone, with active foul smelling discharge +/– bone chips (? sequestrum).
- Healed sinus may be present—may multiple in number.
- Muscle wasting of surrounding muscle

Palpation:
- Widening, broadening with irregularity of affected bone
- With irregular bony margins with deformity with palpable swelling
- Local tenderness +ve

Range of movements: Restricted of nearby joints.

Measurement: True shortening +ve

Provisional diagnosis:

Investigation: Blood, X-ray, CT scan—irregular dead, necrosed, dense bone with pus discharge—send for culture sensitivity.

Summary:

PERTHES DISEASE

(Legg Calve Perthes Disease)
- 4-8 years of age—usual presentation
- Limping without pain
- Restriction of movement of affected hip
- Occasionally pain followed by trivial trauma

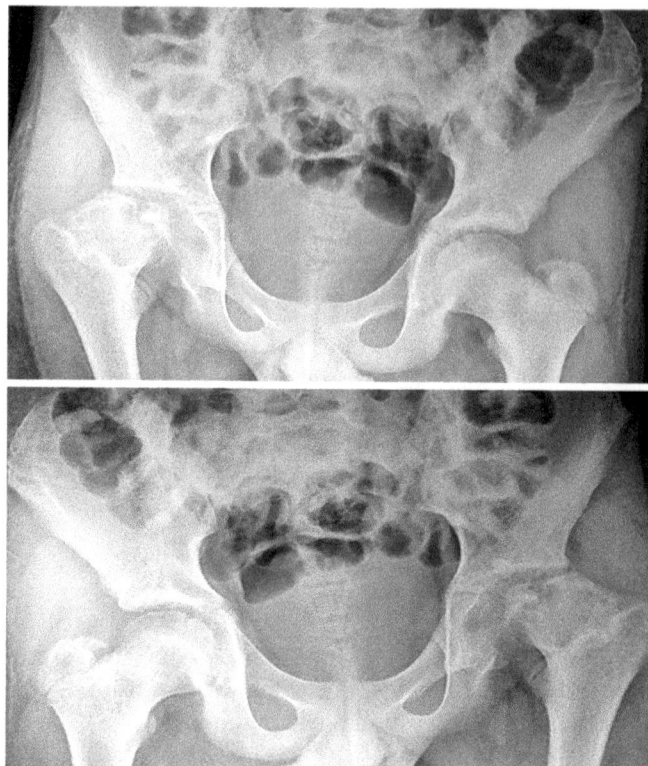

Right femoral head is small, flattened, and fragmented.

- Local tenderness at hip joint line
- Swelling ±ve
- Range of movement—abduction and internal rotation grossly restricted.
- Other movements are normal
- True shortening (0.5-1 cm)

Differential diagnosis:
- *TB hip joint (may occur in child also):*
  - Positive family history (TB)
  - Severe tenderness
  - Adductor spasm will positive in TB hip
  - All movements are restricted
  - Shortening >1-2 cm
  - Constitutional symptoms present
- *Slipped capital femoral epiphysis (SCFE):*
  - Painful limp in tall, thin or short, obese teenage group.
  - No family history
  - No systemic features of tuberculosis
  - Restriction of movement
  - *Transient synovitis:* Gross restriction of all movements.

Pathophysiology of Perthes disease:
- Avascular necrosis of head of femur, in children
- May be followed by trivial trauma
- Venous stasis—arterial occlusion—microcirculation hampered—avascular necrosis (AVN) of head of femur.

Investigation:
- Routine investigation
- X-ray of the both hip
  - Anteroposterior (AP) view
  - Lateral view (must)

Stages (catarrhal classification) radiology based:
- *Type I:* Arterial occlusion stunted (by MRI).
- *Type II:* Fragmentation of head, epiphysis, cyst formation (visible in X-ray).
- *Type III:* Deformed head, followed by coxa magna.
- *Type IV:* Flattening, necrosis of head of femur, followed by subluxation.

Coxa magna—widening and shortening of neck of femur:
- CT scan (CT-guided synovial biopsy)
- MRI (for exact staging)

Treatment of Perthes disease: First confirm stage of the disease

Stage I:
- Bed rest
- Analgesic

Stage II:
- Bed rest
- Analgesic
- Skin traction
- Abduction pillow or abduction brace

Stage III:
- Treatment of stage II
- Corrective osteotomy, e.g., derotation varus osteotomy in proximal femur.

Stage IV:
- Treatment of stage II
- Pelvic osteotomy or Chiari osteotomy

Complication:
- Dislocation may happen in hip
- Shortening
- Secondary osteoarthritis of hip

CARIES SPINE (TB SPINE)

From history:
- Fever, cough, cold
- Family history of TB, past history of TB of patient
- Localized swelling, pain at back with restriction of movement

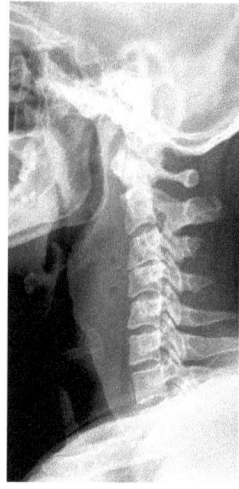

X-ray of cervical spine

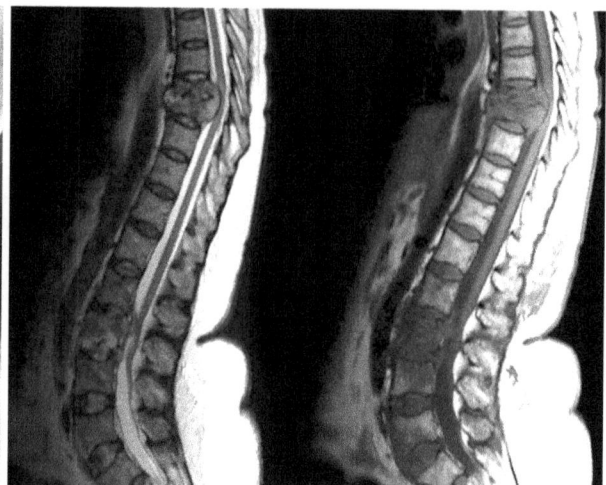

MRI of dorsolateral spine
(affecting both dorsal and lumbar vertebra)

General survey: Pallor ++

Inspection:
- Swelling, Gibbus of dorsal or lumbar spine
- Discharging sinus +ve
- Paraplegia ±, paraparesis ±ve

Palpation:
- Palpation of gibbus
- Palpation of psoas abscess (if any)
- Palpation of regional lymph nodes

Range of movement of spine: Strictly prohibited, do not see or even do not try to see, if you are doing examination of Pott's paraplegia or TB at dorsal or lumbar spine.
- Neurological examination:
    - Higher function
    - Muscle power
    - Muscle tone
    - Reflex
        - Superficial (plantar, abdominal, and cremasteric reflex)
        - Deep jerk (knee, ankle, biceps and triceps jerk)
- Sensory examination

Provisional diagnosis:

Investigation: Blood, X-ray, CT scan, MRI of whole spine.

Summary:

CHAPTER 21

Short Cases

- Nonunion of long bone fracture (#)
- Malunion of long bone fracture
- Chronic osteomyelitis
- Congenital talipes equinovarus (CTEV)
- Cubitus varus/valgus
- Genu varum/valgum
- Foot drop/wrist drop/ulnar claw hand
- Osteosarcoma/Ewing's sarcoma
- Osteochondroma
- Giant cell tumor
- Simple bone cyst/aneurysmal bone cyst

MALUNION

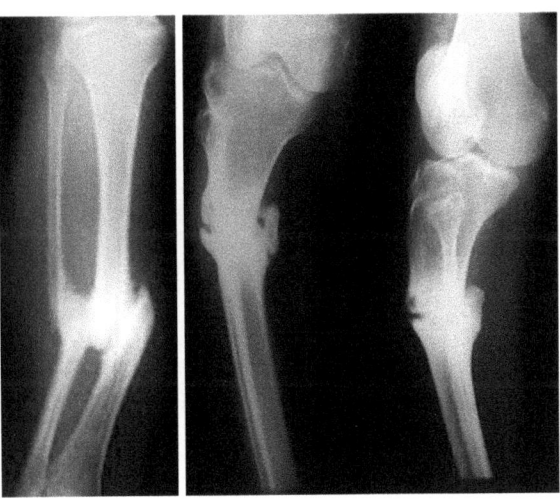

Malunion of fracture both bone leg

Definition: Union in mal-anatomical position

In case of malunited fracture both bone (BB) forearm.

From history:
- History of trauma
- Pain, swelling of M/3 for forearm
- Restricted mobility of affected forearm
- No history of any fever, cough, cold or any drug intake

Clinical examination:
- On inspection:
  - Swelling, deformity of M/3 of affected forearm
  - Visible shortening (if present)
  - Muscle wasting of forearm and sometimes arm, hand muscle
- On palpation—hard, irregular, swelling at M/3 of radial shaft and ulnar shaft, most probably callus.
- Range of motion (ROM) of elbow or wrist joint—if fracture is close to a joint—restricted of movement of that joint.
- Measurement:
  - True shortening +ve
  - Apparent shortening ±ve
- Any other features—any distal neurovascular deficit present or not?

Investigation:
- X-ray of affected forearm with nearby joint—anteroposterior and lateral view.
- Nerve conduction velocity (NCV) study, if suspected nerve injury.

Treatment: Osteoclysis and open reduction + internal fixation (ORIF) by interlocking nail (ILN) or titanium elastic nail (TENS) or limited contact dynamic compression plate (LCDCP) and screws.

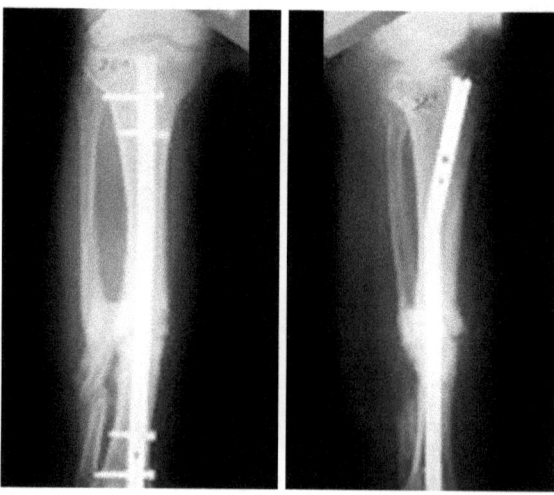

NONUNION

- Nonunion proper—fracture not united >9 months in any long bone.
- Delayed union—fracture not united >6 months time in long bone.
- Un-united fracture—fracture not united >3 months time

Except in fracture neck of femur and fracture scaphoid—where nonunion established by 3 months.

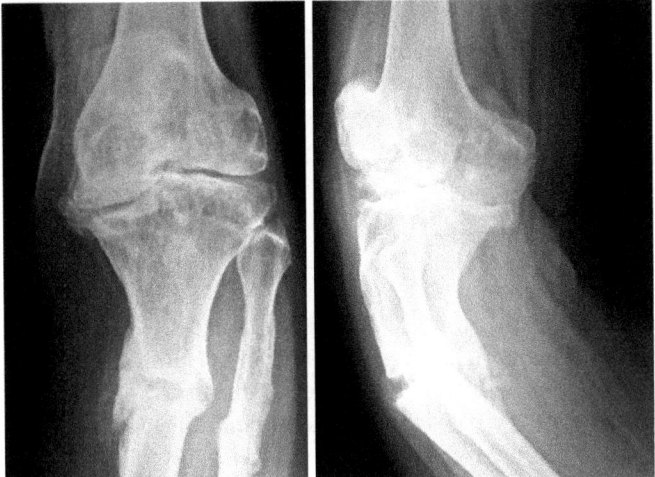

From history: Same like malunion only except (pain ±ve)

Clinical examination:
- Inspection: Same as malunion.
- Palpation:
  - Abnormal mobility at the fracture (fracture) site.
  - Palpable gap may be at fracture site of shaft of long bone (radius or ulnar shaft).
- Others features—same

Treatment:
- Freshening of fracture ends
- Open reduction + internal fixation (ORIF) by TENS or LCDCP with screws.
- Autogenous bone grafting

CUBITUS VARUS

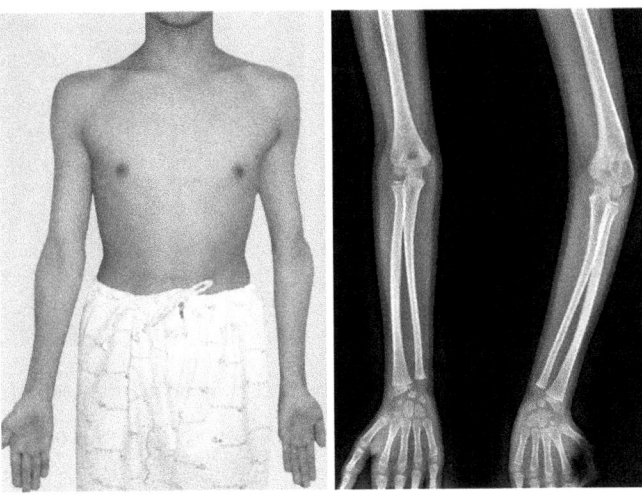

Gunstock deformity due to malunion of any of following fractures:
- Fracture supracondylar humerus (most common)
- Fracture medial condyle of humerus

Point in favor of diagnosis:
- From history: History of trauma in outstretched hand, and may be treated by plaster or indigenous method.
- Inspection: Gunstock deformity at affected elbow with wasting of biceps/triceps/forearm muscle.
- On palpation: No local tenderness
  - Both supracondylar ridges are thickened and broadened
  - Three bony point relationship is maintained (tip of lateral and medial epicondyle and tip of olecranon)—usually form an isosceles triangle.
- Range of movement (ROM) of elbow: If long-standing case—fibrosis of surrounding muscle—causing elbow ROM is restricted—otherwise it is full range (0-140 degree).
- True shortening of arm: Positive (from tip of acromion angle of scapula to tip of lateral epicondyle) (alternative arm length measurement process—tip of olecranon process, if lateral epicondyle is fractured).

Investigation: X-ray of elbow—anteroposterior and lateral view.

Treatment: After measurement of Bowmann's angle—modified French osteotomy.

Note: In case of fracture malunited fracture medial condyle with cubitus varus all findings are same except on palpation—only medial supracondylar ridge will be thickened and broadened.

CUBITUS VALGUS

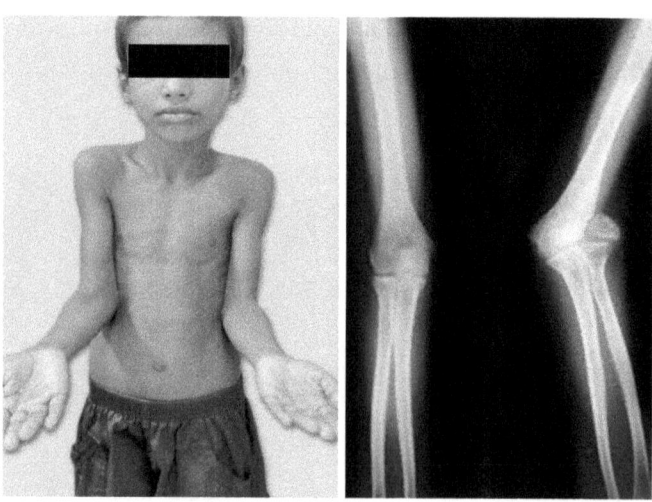

X-ray of fracture lateral condyle with cubitus valgus (right side)

Deformity due to malunion of fracture lateral condyle (most common) or malunion of fracture supracondylar humerus.

All findings same except on:
- **Inspection:** Elbow deviated laterally and carrying angle is more than normal
- **Palpation:** Lateral supracondylar ridge thickened, broadened
- **Treatment:** Corrective osteotomy
- **Complication:** Tardy ulnar nerve palsy

FOOT DROP

Etiology:
- Traumatic injury to common peroneal nerve at knee injury (common site)
- Leprosy
- Any neurological disorder (like diabetic peripheral neuropathy)

Clinical examination:
- On inspection:
  - Affected foot is plantar fixed.
  - Wasting of calf and foot muscle
  - Swelling of foot ±ve
  - Shiny skin on dorsum of foot
- On palpation:
  - In traumatic injury—cut mark on skin at the fibular neck or around may be present
  - In Leprosy or other neurological disorders—nerve is thickened at nerve of fibula
- ROM of ankle joint: Active dorsiflexion is not possible.
- Neurological test:
  - Motor—tone of foot muscle is decreased
  - Sensory deficit—at ankle and foot (plantar/dorsum aspect)

Investigation:
- X-ray of affected knee—anteroposterior and lateral view.
- NCV studies of the lower limb

Treatment:
- Observation
- Foot drop splint
- Operative: Tendon transfer of tibialis posterior to midtarsal region

WRIST DROP

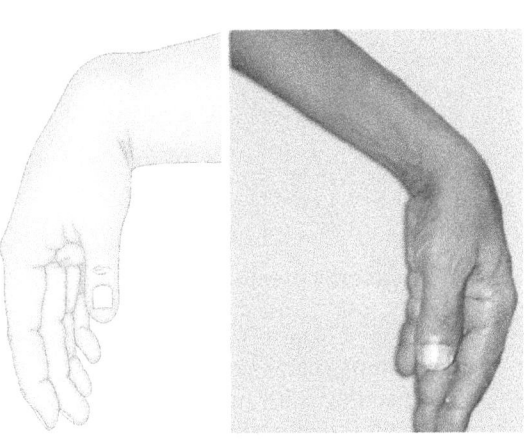

Etiology: Due to radial nerve palsy.

Clinical examination:
- History of injury to arm by road traffic accident (RTA) with inability to extend wrist.

- On inspection:
  - In ability to do dorsiflexion of wrist actively
  - Wasting of forearm/wrist muscle
  - Shiny skin of forearm/wrist
  - Swelling of hand or wrist ±ve
- On palpation: Malunited or nonunion fracture shaft of humerus present with a swelling at fracture site.
- Range of movement:
  - Shoulder and elbow—full range only
  - Wrist dorsiflexion (active)—0 degree
  - Wrist palmar flexion—active is possible 0–50 degree flexion.
- Neurological examination:
  - Muscle tone of forearm/hand muscle
  - Brachioradialis jerk—absent
  - Sensory examination—deficit present below the level of nerve injury or entrapment

Treatment:
- Observation
- Fracture stabilization by open reduction + internal fixation (ORIF) with interlocking nail (ILN) or by limited contact dynamic compression plate (LCDCP) or LCP
- Dynamic cock-up splint
- If no recovery—tendon transfer

ULNAR CLAW HAND

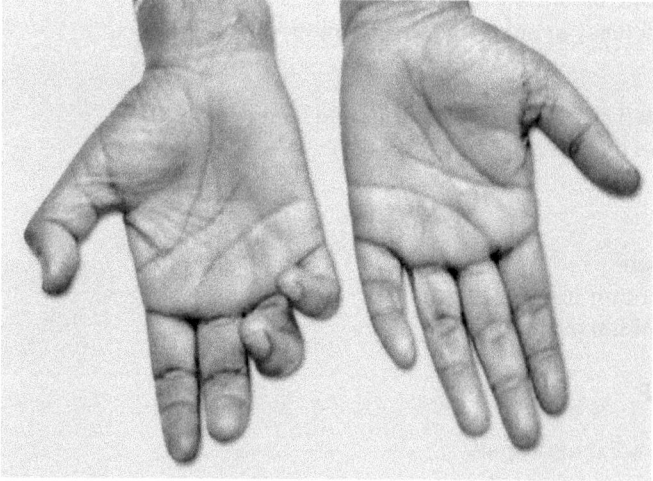

It is due to ulnar nerve injury.

Clinical features:
- From history: History of injury to elbow
- On inspection: Clawing of ring and little finger of affected hand, wasting of hypothenar muscle, and interossei.

- On palpation:
  - Thickening of ulnar nerve behind medial epicondyle
  - Finger abduction—is weak, loss of thumb adduction
- Neurological examination: Tone of hypothenar muscle, card test +ve
- Froment's sign +ve (due weakness of adductor pollicis)

Treatment:
- Observation
- Stabilization of metacarpophalangeal (MCP) joint in flexion by flexor digitorum superficialis tendon transfer.
- Restoration for index abduction by extensor tendon transfer to dorsal 1st interossei.

GENU VARUM

Commonest cause:
- In child—rickets
- In adult:
  - Osteoarthritis (>50 years)
  - Rheumatoid arthritis (in female)

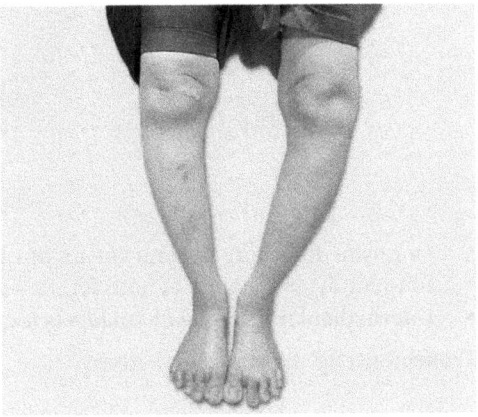

Clinical sign: On inspection—both leg deformed toward midline, i.e., bowed [intercondylar distance of both femur (normal) is 4-6 cm and intermalleolar distance in ankle is (normal 6-8 cm)].

Clinical features of rickets:
- Craniotabes
- Thickening of knee, ankle, wrist, from epiphyseal overgrowth
- Rickety rosary
- Harrison's sulcus
- Genu varum/valgum
- Coxa vara ±ve with fractures of bone.

Investigation:
- X-ray:
  - Thickening, widening, cupping of metaphysis and epiphysis
  - Incomplete stress fracture
  - Trefoil pelvis (lateral indentation of acetabulum)
- Blood:
  - Calcium, phosphate, and alkaline phosphatase
  - In vitamin D deficiency—25 HCC is decreased
- Bone biopsy

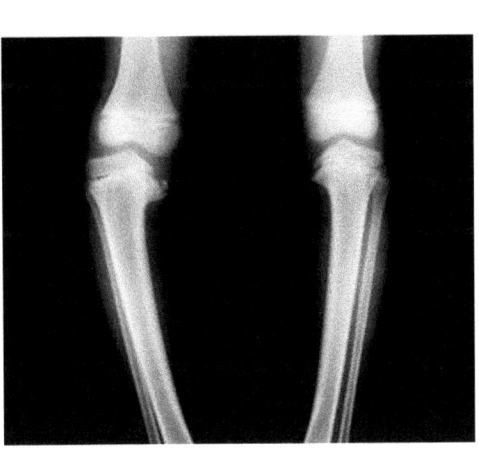

Treatment: If deformity due to rickets—treatment of rickets or any other cause and operative by corrective osteotomy.

GENU VALGUM

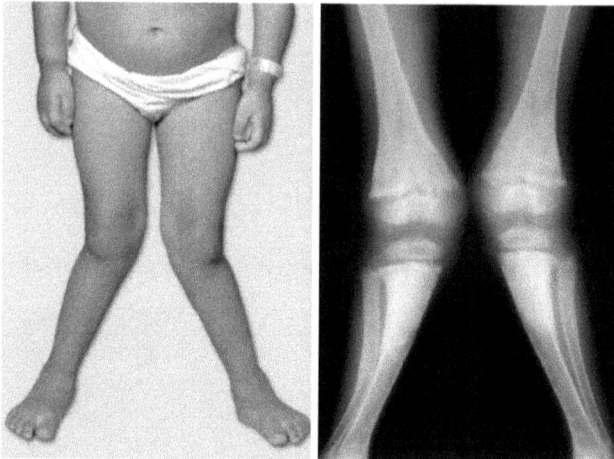

A case of rickets

- Opposite deformity to genu varum or in short called knock knee
- Intercondylar distance of both femur—is decreased
- Intermalleolar distance of ankle—is increased

Treatment: By corrective osteotomy.

CHAPTER 22

Operative

Tension band wiring (TBW): Already mentioned in fracture olecranon treatment.
Tension band wiring (TBW): Already mentioned in fracture patella treatment.

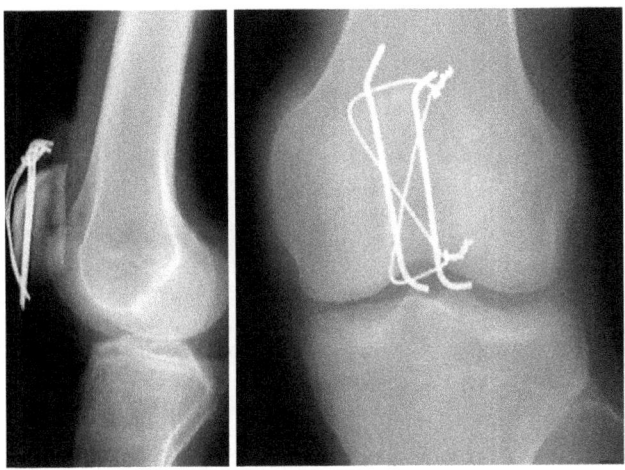

K-NAIL IN FRACTURE SHAFT OF FEMUR (FRACTURE SOF)

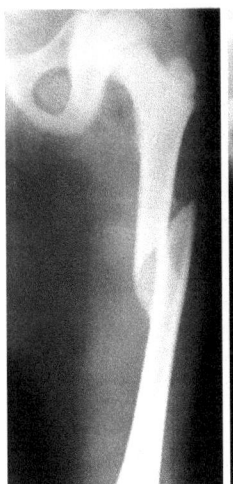
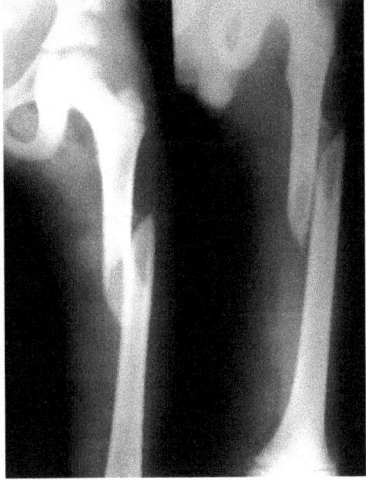
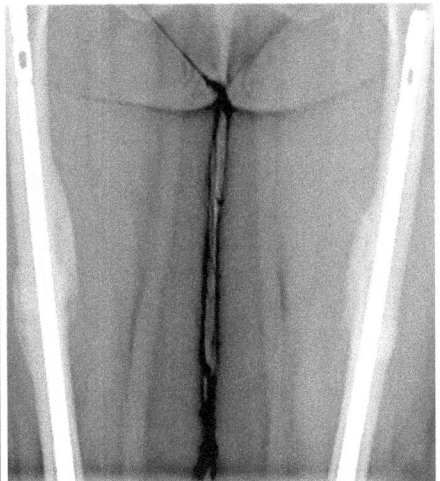

Preoperative X-ray of fracture shaft of femur

Postoperative X-ray of fracture shaft of femur with K-nail

Procedure:
- Under anesthesia (mostly regional) in lateral position
- After aseptic dressing/draping
- Lateral approach to fracture site—incision given a line joining greater trochanter tip and lateral condyle of femur.
- Tensor fasciae latae cut
- Vastus lateralis splitting done
- Fracture exposed and look for fracture anatomy
- Open reduction by two reduction forceps and hold it by Lowmann's clamp
- Internal fixation by K-nail (antegrade/retrograde)
- Wash with normal saline (NS)
- Wound closed is layers
- Atrial septal defect (ASD) done

PLATE FIXATION IN FRACTURE SHAFT OF FEMUR

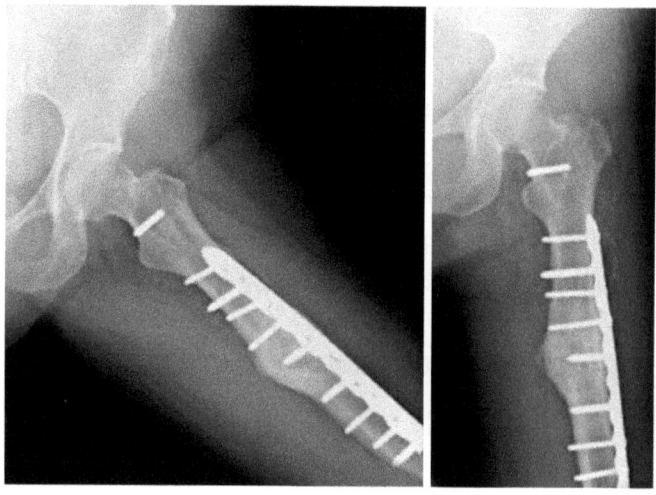

Same like K-nail in fracture shaft of femur (SOF)—up to open reduction and then:
- Internal fixation by 4.5 mm limited contact dynamic compression plate (LCDCP) with cortical screws
- Wash with NS
- Wound closed in layers
- ASD done
- Derotation shoe given

PLATE FIXATION IN FRACTURE BOTH BONE FOREARM

After open reduction and:
- Internal fixation by 3.5 mm limited contact dynamic compression plate (LCDCP) with cortical screws

Operative

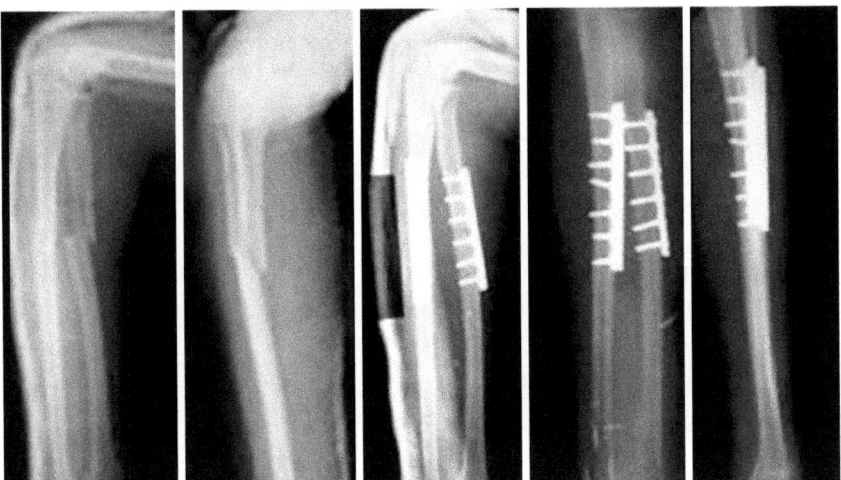

- Wash with NS
- Wound closed in layers
- ASD done

CHAPTER 23

Instruments

SCREW DRIVER

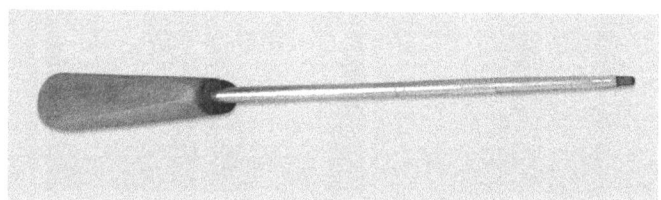

Use: For using screw in limited contact dynamic compression plate (LCDCP) in internal fixation of fracture shaft of femur (SOF), both bone forearm after open reduction.

Sterilization: By autoclaving (temperature—121°C, pressure—15-20 lb/sq inch, time—30 minutes.

PERIOSTEUM ELEVATOR

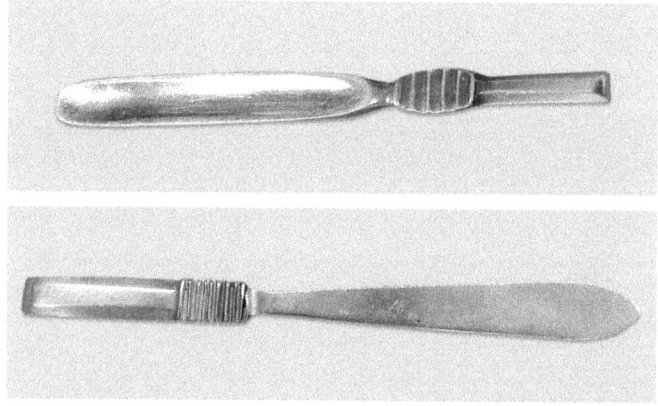

Use: For using elevation of periosteum in any open reduction and internal fixation of fracture SOF, both bone forearm.

Sterilization: By autoclaving (temperature—121°C, pressure—15-20 lb/sq inch, time—30 minutes.

BONE PLIERS

Use: For cutting K-wire and S-S wire, used in any orthopedic surgery like open reduction + internal fixation (ORIF) with tension band wiring (TBW) for fracture patella.

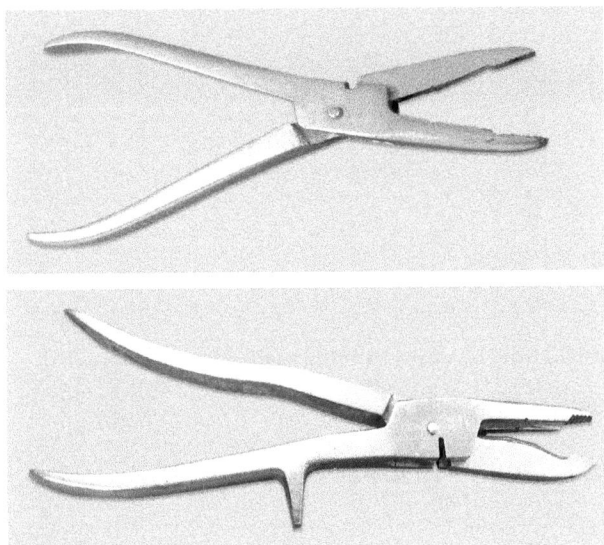

Sterilization: By autoclaving.

BONE CHISEL—ONE END IS BEVELLED

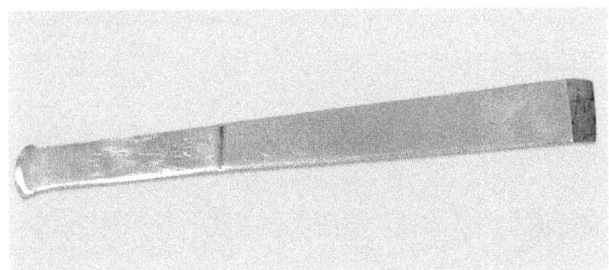

Use: For osteotomy in malunion and Perthes disease and saucerization in chronic osteomylitis.

Sterilization: By autoclaving.

SEQUESTRECTOMY FORCEP—SINGLE HINGE

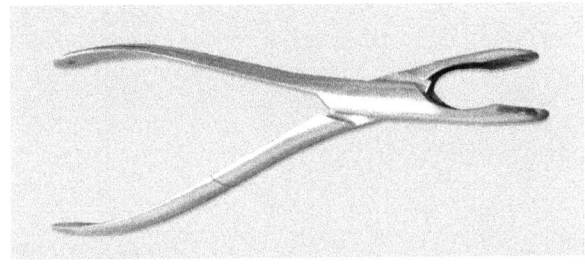

Use: For sequestrectomy and saucerization in chronic osteomylitis.

Sterilization: By autoclaving.

BONE TAP

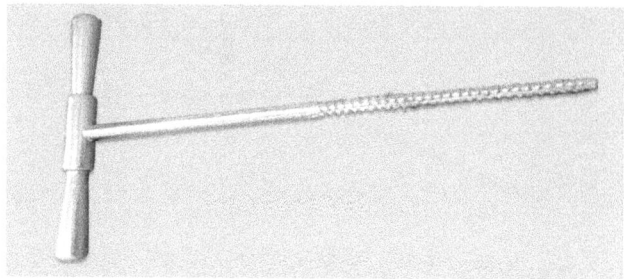

Use: For tapping the drill hole in screw or bone plate fixation after ORIF.

Sterilization: By autoclaving.

BONE CUTTING FORCEP—DOUBLE HINGE

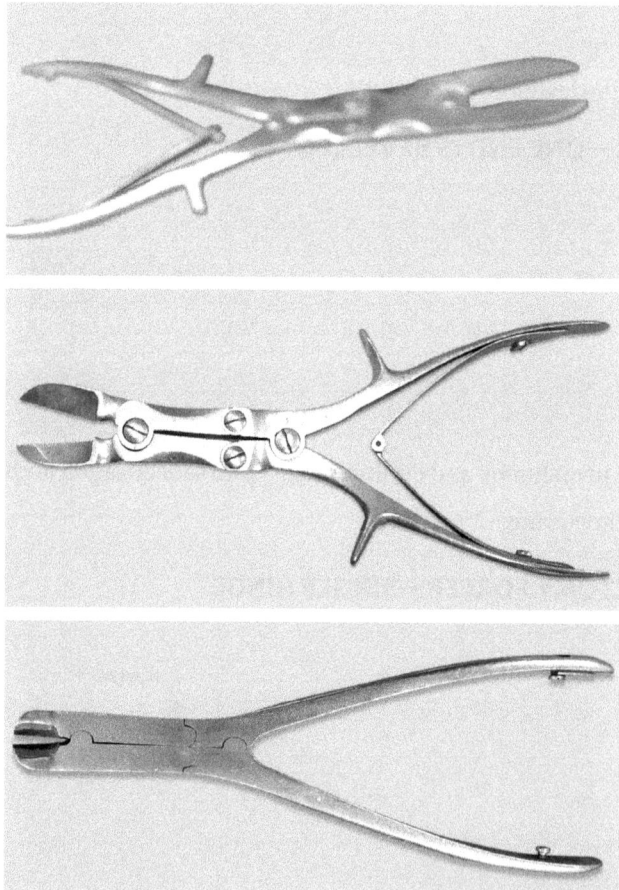

Use: For osteotomy at the level of phalanx and metacarpal and metatarsal bone.

Sterilization: By autoclaving.

BONE NIBBLER

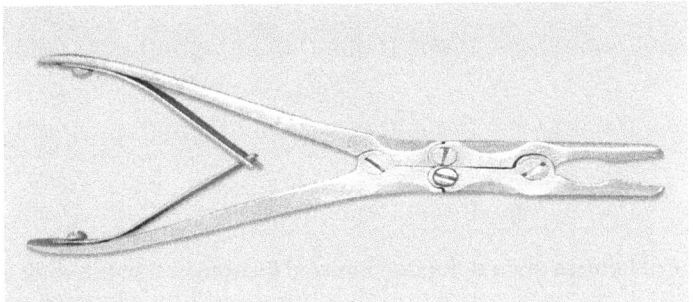

Use: For nibbling of bone in nonunion of fracture and in tumor surgery.

Sterilization: By autoclaving.

BONE LEVER (BRISTOW'S)

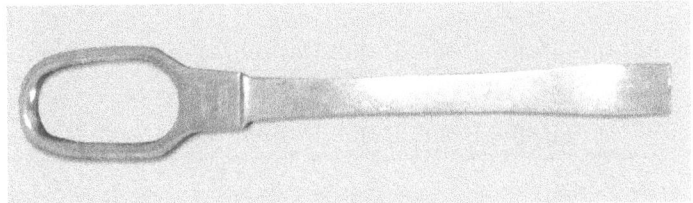

Use: For leverage of bone in open reduction internal fixation in fracture shaft of femur.

Sterilization: By autoclaving.

BONE LEVER—POINTED

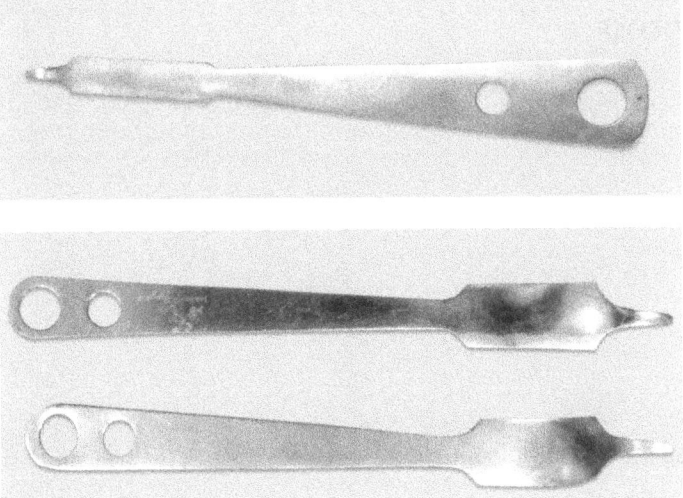

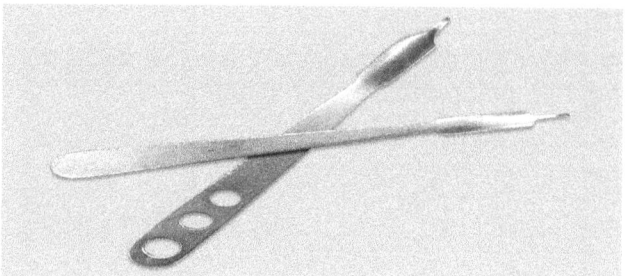

Use: For leverage of bone in open reduction internal fixation in fracture shaft of femur.

Sterilization: By autoclaving.

ALLIS TISSUE FORCEPS

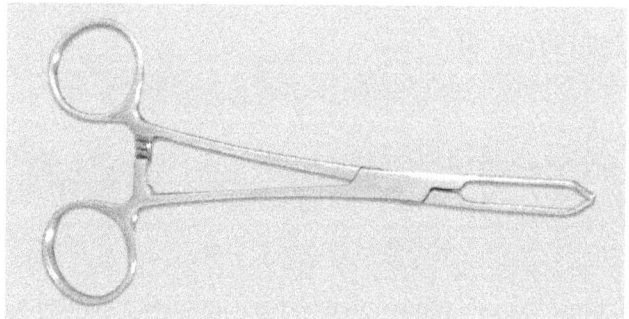

Use: For holding deep fascia during dissection open reduction internal fixation in fracture shaft of femur.

Sterilization: By autoclaving.

NEEDLE HOLDER

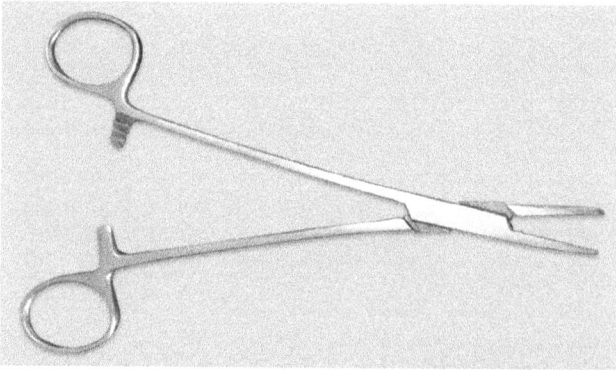

Use: For suturing the wound after end of surgery with the help of a needle & slik.

Sterilization: By autoclaving.

BONE CURETTE

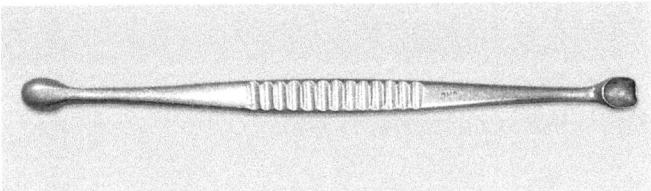

Use: For curettage of bony cavity, freshening of fracture ends in nonunion, during the debridement in chronic osteomyelitis.

Sterilization: By autoclaving.

HEMOSTATIC FORCEPS

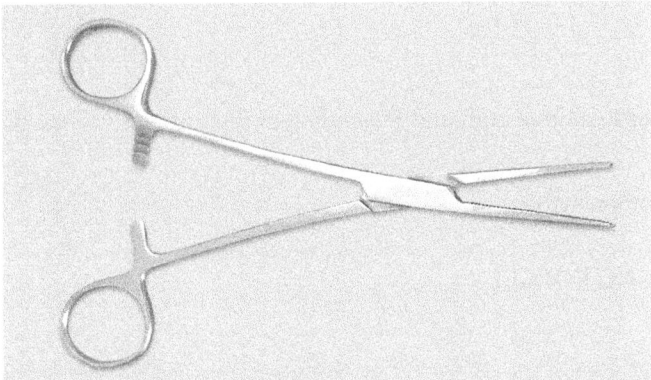

Use: For catching bleeding blood vessel during open reduction internal fixation.

Sterilization: By autoclaving.

BONE GOUGE

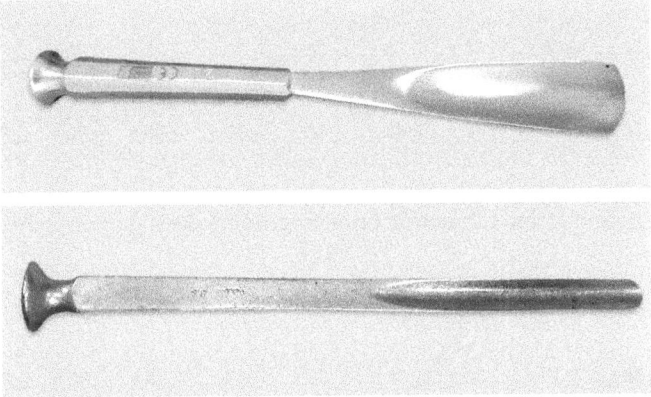

Use: For taking cancellous bone graft and freshening of fracture ends in fracture nonunion.

Sterilization: By autoclaving.

OSTEOTOME

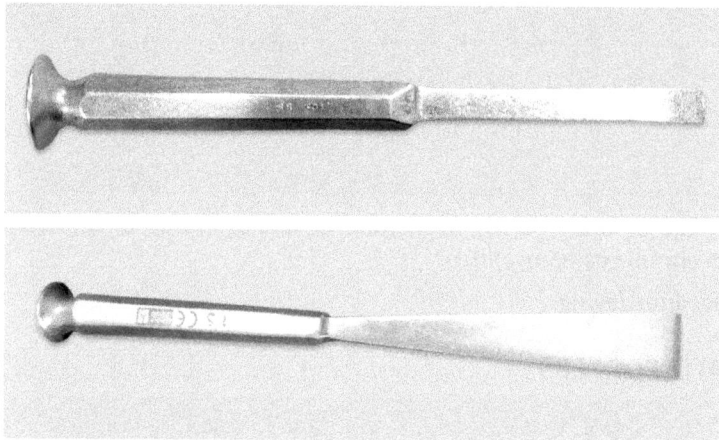

Use: For taking cortical bone graft and freshening of fracture ends in fracture nonunion and osteotomy of bone.

Sterilization: By autoclaving.

BONE HOLDING FORCEP

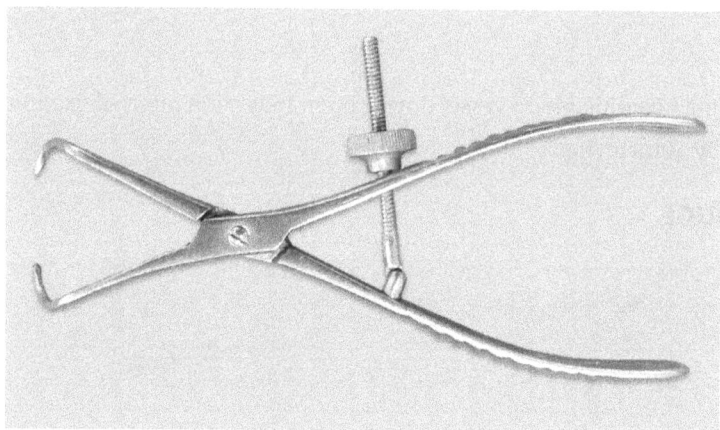

Use: For holding the reduction of fracture bony fragments during open reduction and internal frication.

Sterilization: By autoclaving.

MALLET/HAMMER

Use: Along with osteotome for taking cortical bone graft and freshening of fracture ends in fracture nonunion and osteotomy of bone.

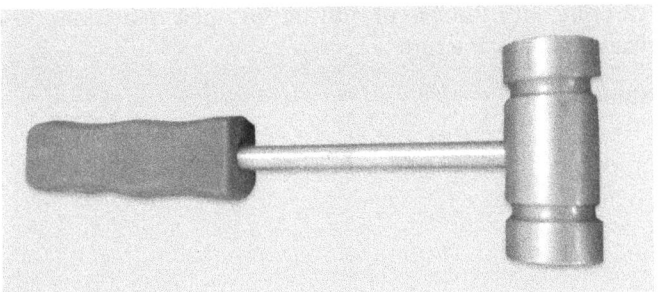

Sterilization: By autoclaving.

RIMMER

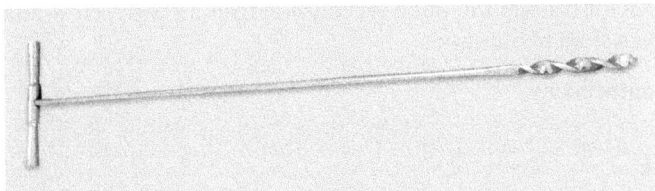

Use: For rimming before introduction of K-nail in fracture shaft of femur after open reduction.

Sterilization: By autoclaving.

CANNULATED RIMMER

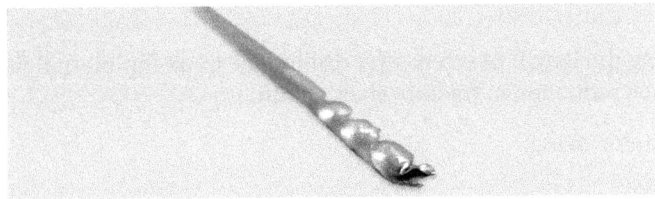

Use: For rimming before introduction of Interlocking nail in fracture shaft of femur after open reduction.

Sterilization: By autoclaving.

MANNMANN ELECTRIC DRILL HAND PIECE WITH KEY

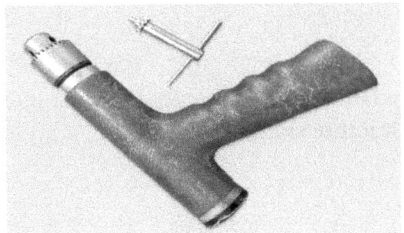

Use: For drilling of bone with the use of drill bit for open reduction/close reduction with internal/external fixation in any fracture.

Sterilization: By autoclaving.

DRILL BIT

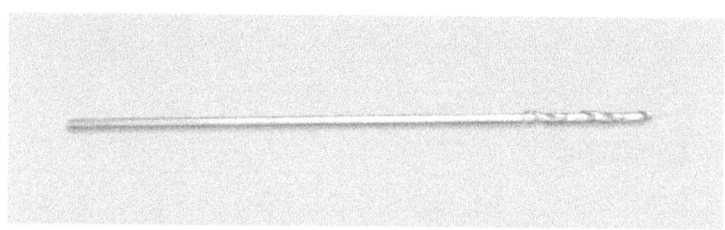

Use: Used with drill for drilling the bone for internal fixation with screw and plate after open reduction in fracture shaft of humerus.

Sterilization: By autoclaving.

DEPTH GAZE

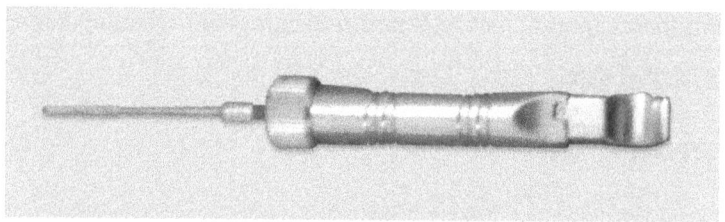

Use: For measuring the length of screw after drilling the bone for internal fixation with screw and plate after open reduction in fracture shaft of humerus.

Sterilization: By autoclaving.

DRILL GUIDE

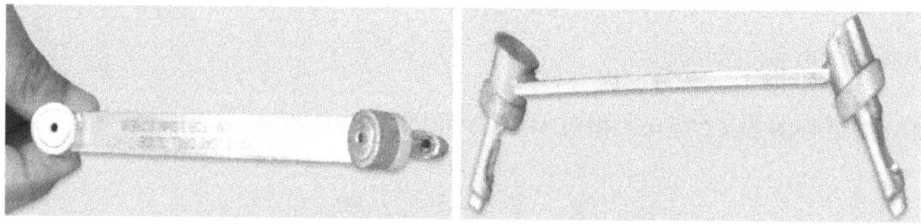

Use: Used with drill bit as guidance for drilling the bone for internal fixation with screw and plate after open reduction in fracture shaft of humerus.

Sterilization: By autoclaving.

IMPACTER

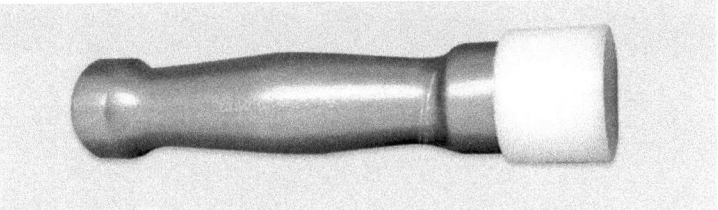

Use: Used for impaction of prosthesis in hemiarthroplasty in fracture neck of femur.

Sterilization: By autoclaving.

PATELLA HOLDING FORCEP

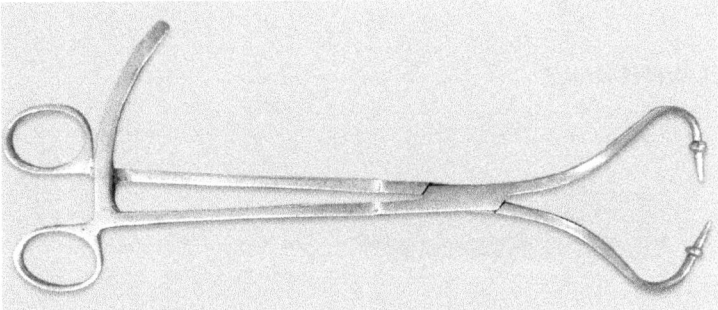

Use: Holding the fracture fragments of patella during open reduction and internal fixation with tension band wiring for fracture patella.

Sterilization: By autoclaving.

LANGENBECK'S RETRACTOR

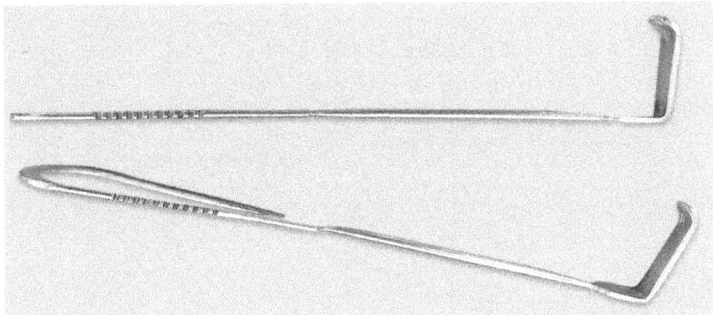

Use: Retraction of the deepseated muscle during open reduction and internal fixation for any long bone fracture.

Sterilization: By autoclaving.

BONE HOLDING FORCEPS

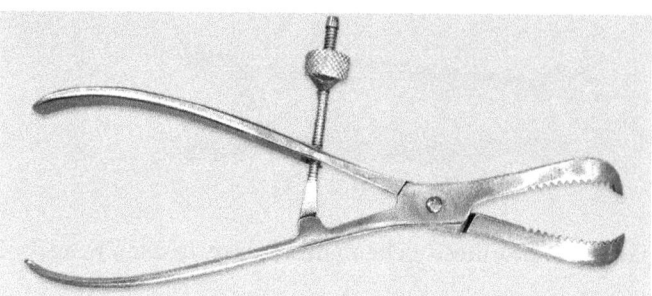

Use: For holding the fracture fragments of long bone during open reduction and internal/external fixation for any long bone fracture.

Sterilization: By autoclaving.

BONE AWL WITH HOLE

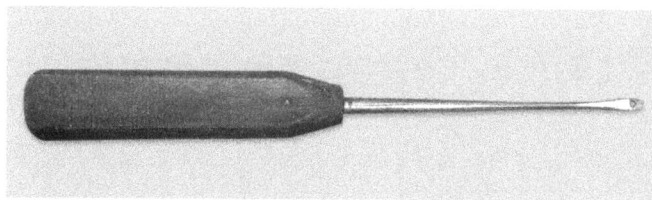

Use: For passing stainless steel wire in tension band wiring in fracture patella or long bone fracture during open reduction and internal/external fixation.

Sterilization: By autoclaving.

PLATE HOLDING FORCEPS

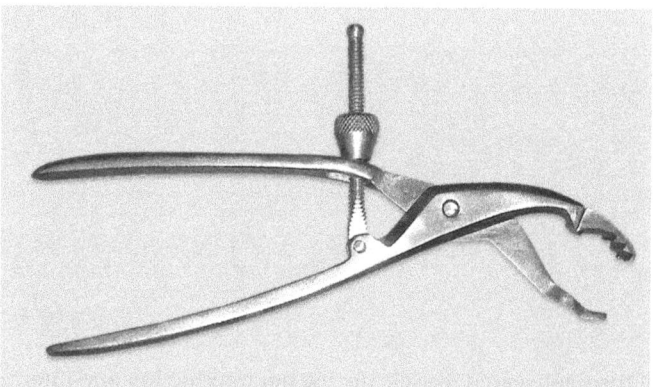

Use: For holding fracture fragments with plate during reduction, in open reduction and internal fixation for long bone fracture.

Sterilization: By autoclaving.

LOWMANNS BONE HOLDING CLAMP

Use: For holding fracture fragments with plate after reduction during open reduction and internal/external fixation.

Sterilization: By autoclaving.

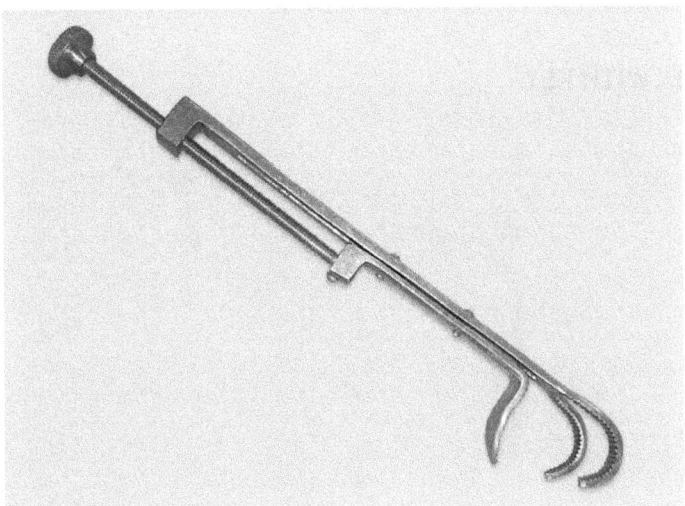

T HANDLE FOR PIN INTRODUCTION

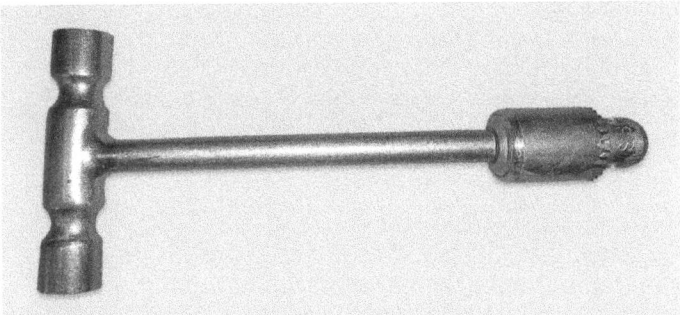

Use: For holding Schanz pin during introduction into the drill hold of long bone during open reduction and external fixation, during gross degloving injury of hand/foot, or any long bone open fracture.

Sterilization: By autoclaving.

SPANNER WRENCH FOR EXTERNAL FIXATOR

Use: For tightening the nuts of universal clamp with Schanz pin during open reduction and external fixation, during gross degloving injury of hand/foot, or any long bone open fracture.

Sterilization: By autoclaving.

Instruments

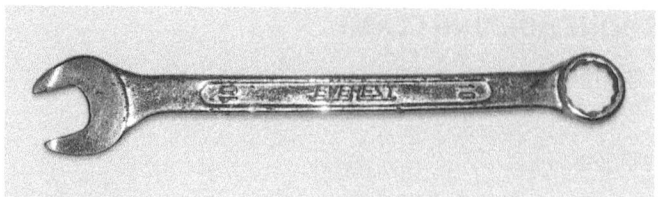

HAND DRILL WITH KEY

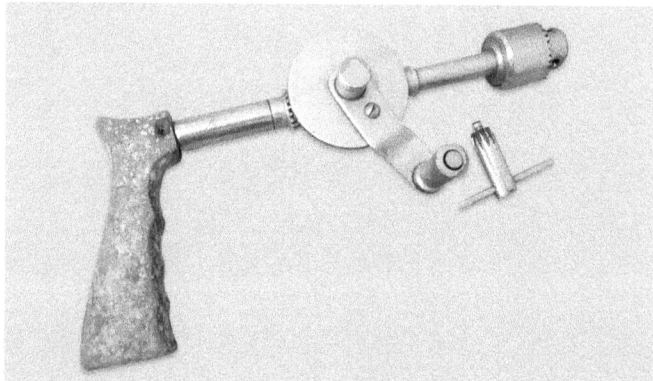

Use: For drilling the bone manually with help of drill bit in any fixation for long bone fracture or short bone fracture during open reduction and external/internal fixation.

Sterilization: By autoclaving.

CHAPTER 24

Implants

AUSTIN MOORE PROSTHESIS

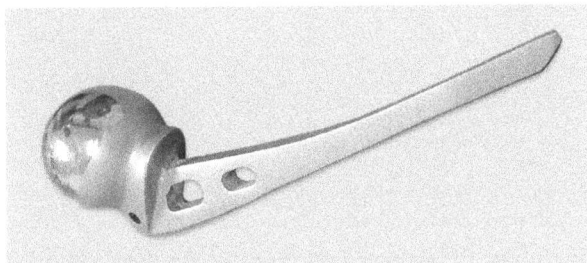

Use: Hemiarthroplasty in fracture neck of femur (NOF).

Sterilization:
- Usually prosthesis is available in sterile pack.
- If not sterile pack available then by autoclaving.

BIPOLAR PROSTHESIS

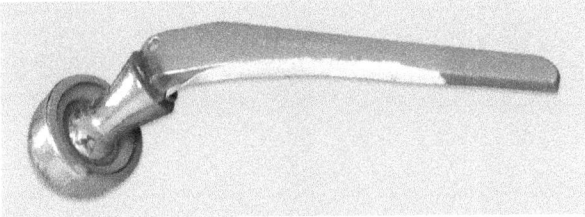

Use: Hemiarthroplasty in fracture neck of femur.

Sterilization:
- Usually prosthesis is available in sterile pack.
- If not sterile pack available then by autoclaving.

STEINMANN PIN (4.5 MM)

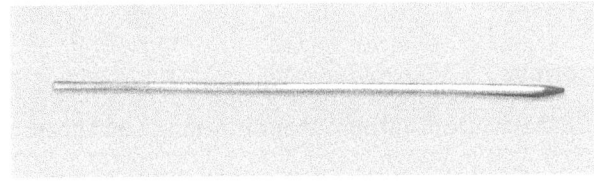

Use: Skeletal traction (upper tibial/lower femoral) in fracture trochanter, fracture shaft of femur.

Sterilization: By autoclaving.

STEINMANN PIN WITH BHOLER'S STIRRUP

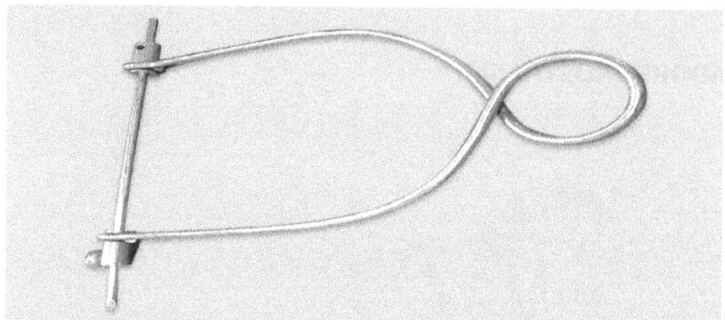

Use: Skeletal traction (upper tibial/lower femoral) in fracture trochanter, fracture shaft of femur.

Sterilization: By autoclaving.

CORTICAL SCREW

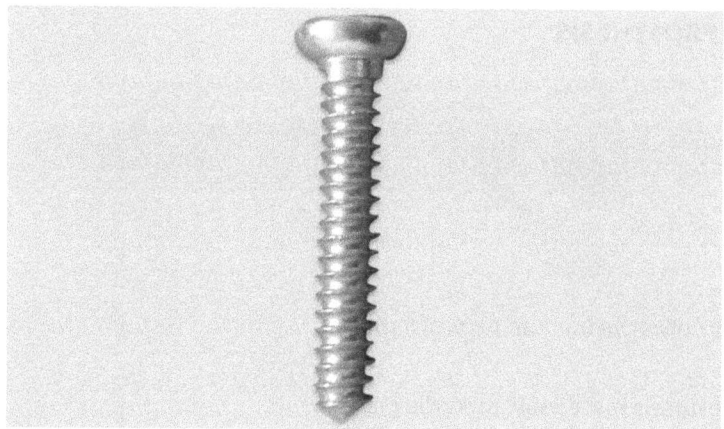

Use: With dynamic compression plate (DCP)/ limited contact dynamic compression plate (LCDCP) in fracture both bone forearm, fracture shaft of humerus for internal fixation.

Sterilization: By autoclaving.

CANCELLOUS SCREW

Use: With DCP/LCDCP in fracture distal humerus, distal femur and fracture proximal humerus for internal fixation.

Sterilization: By autoclaving.

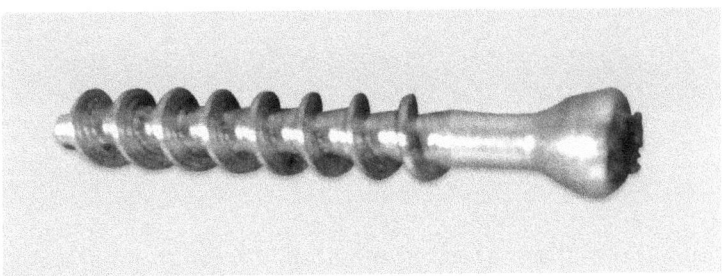

LIMITED CONTACT DYNAMIC COMPRESSION PLATE

Use: For internal fixation in fracture shaft of femur, fracture both bone forearm, fracture shaft of humerus, after open reduction.

Sterilization: By autoclaving.

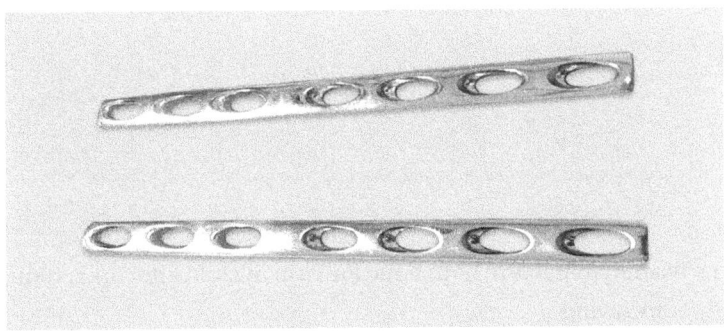

K-NAIL

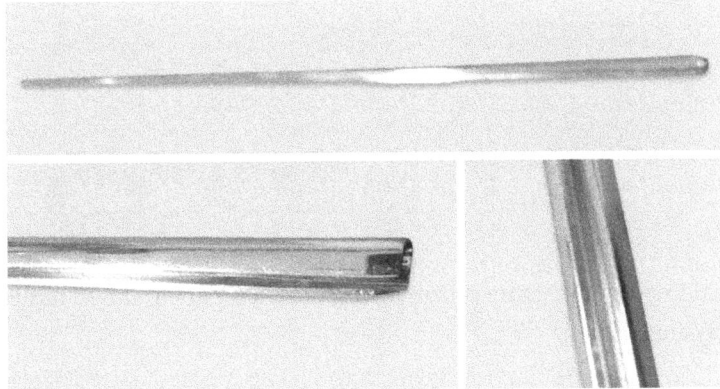

Use: For internal fixation in fracture shaft of femur, can be used in fracture shaft of tibia also, after open reduction.

Sterilization: By autoclaving.

K-WIRE

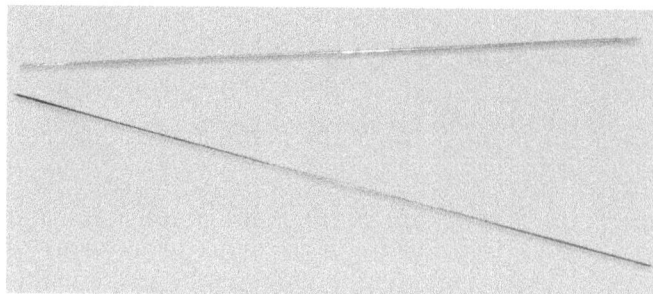

Use: In percutaneous pinning in supracondylar fracture humerus in child, after closed reduction. Also used in metacarpal fracture or metatarsal fracture fixation after open reduction.
Sterilization: By autoclaving.

RUSH NAIL

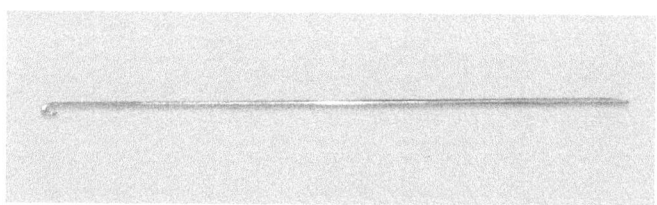

Use: For internal fixation in fracture both bone forearm in child after open reduction.
Sterilization: By autoclaving.

PHILOS PLATE

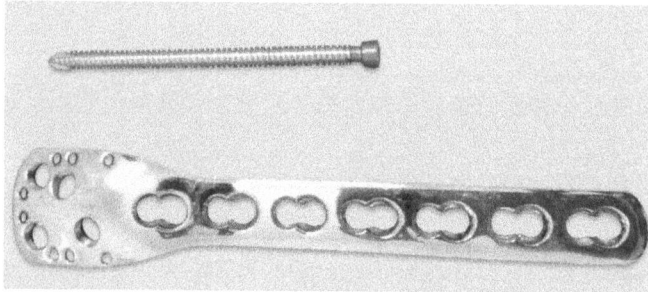

Use: For internal fixation in fracture proximal humerus, after open/closed reduction.
Sterilization: By autoclaving.

RECONSTRUCTION PLATE

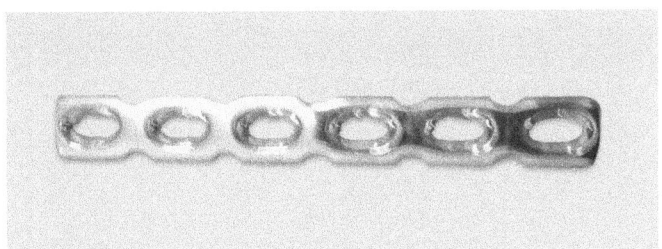

Use: For internal fixation in fracture distal humerus and fracture acetabulum, after open reduction.

Sterilization: By autoclaving.

DYNAMIC HIP SCREW WITH BARREL PLATE

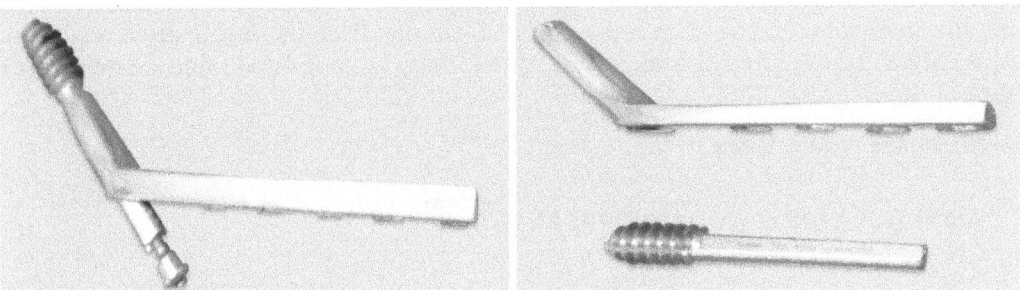

Use: For internal fixation in fracture intertrochanteric femur after close reduction under image guidance.

Sterilization: By autoclaving.

DISTAL FEMORAL LOCKING PLATE

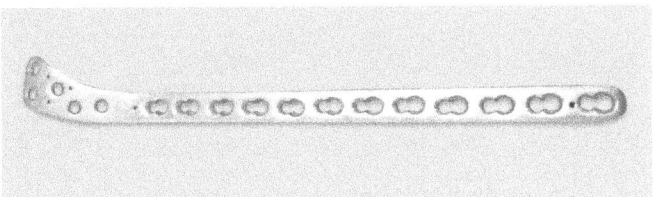

Use: For internal fixation in fracture distal femur with intra-articular extension, after close/open reduction under image guidance.

Sterilization: By autoclaving.

DISTRACTOR OF EXTERNAL FIXATOR WITH ALLEN KEY

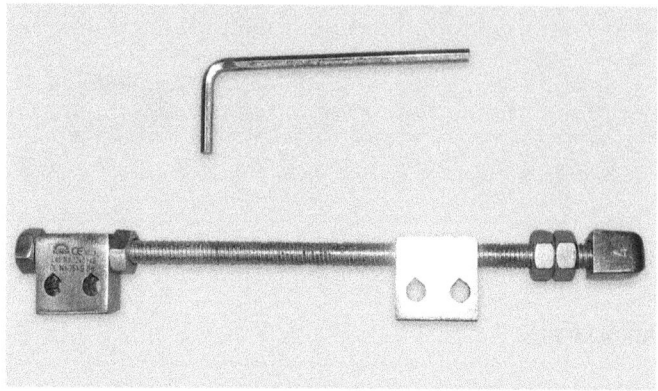

Use: For holding fracture fragments with K-wire (passing through bone), or small Schanz pin after reduction during open reduction and external fixation, during gross degloving injury of hand/foot, or for the correction of deformity in congenital talipes equinovarus (CTEV).

Sterilization: By autoclaving.

AO TUBULAR ROD AND UNIVERSAL CLAMP

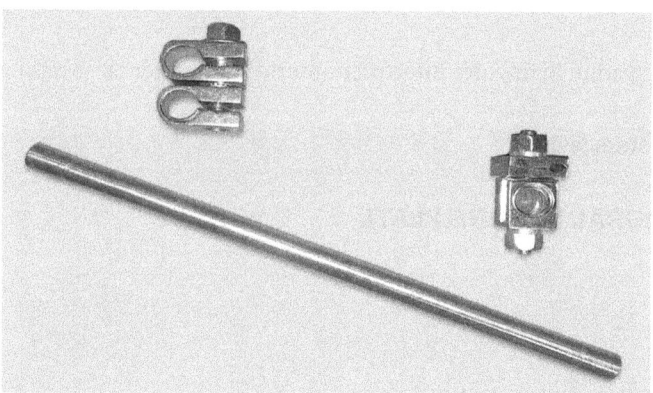

Use: For fix the fracture fragments of long bone during open reduction and external fixation for any long bone open fracture.

Sterilization: By autoclaving.

SCHANZ PIN

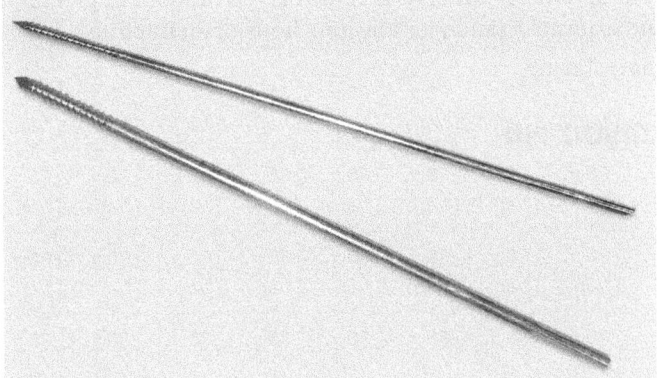

Use: For holding the fracture fragments (minimum two pins on each side of fracture) of long bone during open reduction and external fixation for any long bone open fracture.

Sterilization: By autoclaving.

CORTICAL AND CANCELLOUS SCHANZ PIN

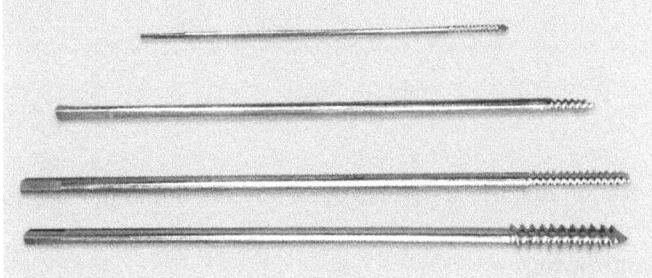

Use: For holding the fracture fragments (minimum two pins on each side of fracture) of long bone during open reduction and external fixation for any long bone open fracture.

Sterilization: By autoclaving.

CANCELLOUS SCHANZ PIN

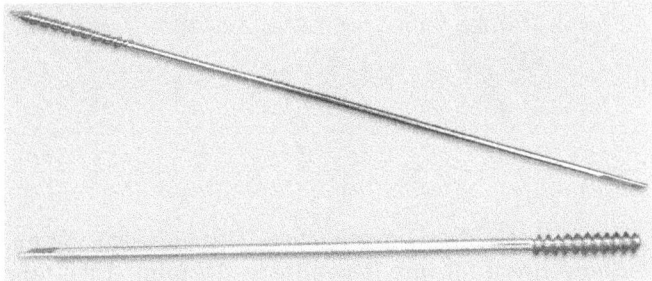

Use: For holding the fracture fragments (minimum two pins on each side of fracture) of cancellous part of long bone or cancellous bone like calcaneum or greater trochanter during open reduction and external fixation for any long bone open fracture.

Sterilization: By autoclaving.

CORTICAL SCHANZ PIN

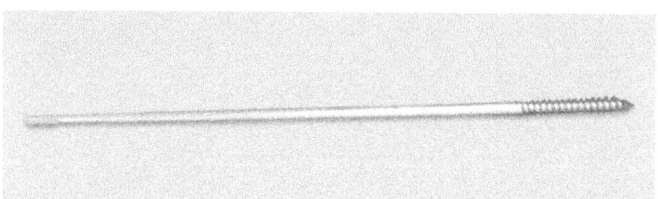

Use: For external fixation in cortical bone in open fracture both bone leg and fracture pelvis, after open reduction.

Sterilization: By autoclaving.

CORTICAL SCHANZ PIN WITH UNIVERSAL CLAMP

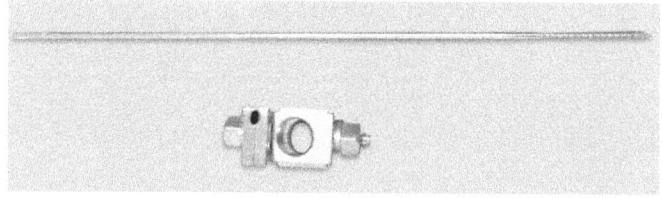

Use: For external fixation in cortical bone in open fracture both bone leg and fracture pelvis, after open reduction.

Sterilization: By autoclaving.

UNIVERSAL CLAMP WITH T-CLAMP AND TUBE-TUBE CLAMP

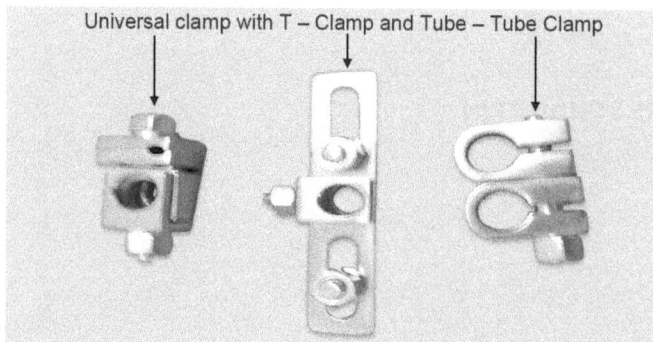

Universal clamp with T – Clamp and Tube – Tube Clamp

Use: For external fixation assembly in open fracture both bone leg and fracture pelvis, after open reduction. T-clamp use if fracture is nearby to the joint. Tube-tube clamp used for connecting two tubes.

Sterilization: By autoclaving.

AO TUBULAR ROD WITH UNIVERSAL CLAMP

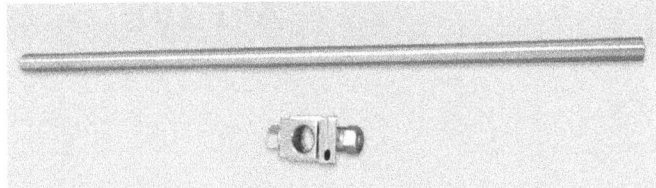

Use: For external fixation in open fracture both bone leg and fracture pelvis, after open reduction.

Sterilization: By autoclaving.

K-NAIL WITH RIMMER (BELOW)

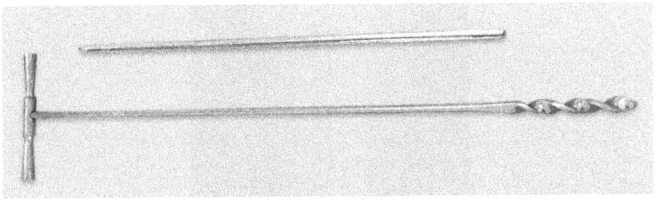

Use: K-nail used for internal fixation for fracture shaft of femur.

Sterilization: By autoclaving.

CHAPTER 25

X-rays

X-RAY OF FRACTURE BOTH BONE LEG (FRACTURE TIBIA DISTAL 1/3RD, AND FIBULA UPPER 1/3RD)

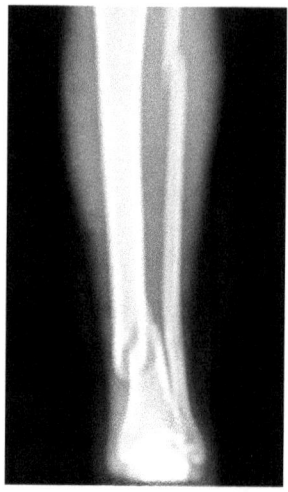

Treatment: By close reduction and internal fixation (CRIF) by interlocking nail.

X-RAY OF FRACTURE SUPRACONDYLAR HUMERUS IN A CHILD

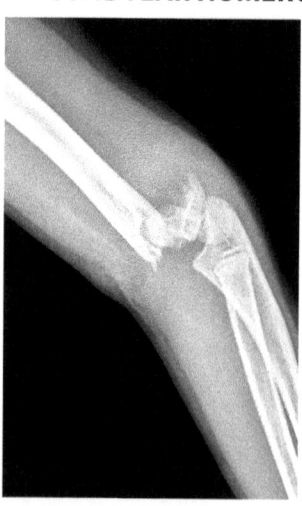

Treatment: By closed reduction and two parallel or cris-cross K-wire/percutaneous pin under image guidance.

X-RAY OF FRACTURE PELVIS

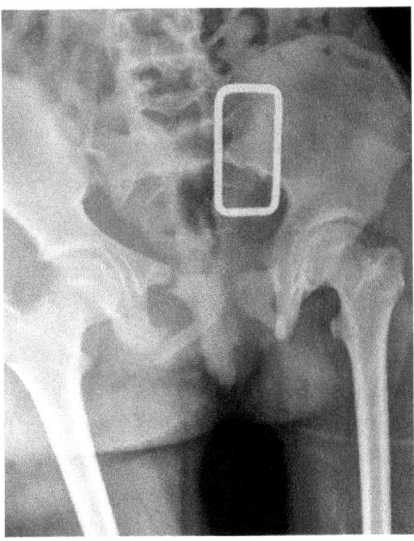

Treatment: By closed reduction and external fixation.

X-RAY OF FRACTURE SHAFT OF DISTAL FEMUR IN CHILD

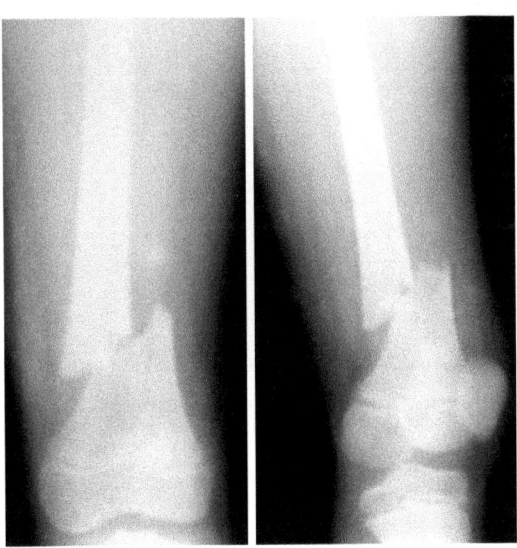

Treatment: By closed reduction and internal fixation (CRIF) by titanium elastic nail system (TENS).

X-RAY OF FRACTURE SHAFT OF FEMUR IN A CHILD

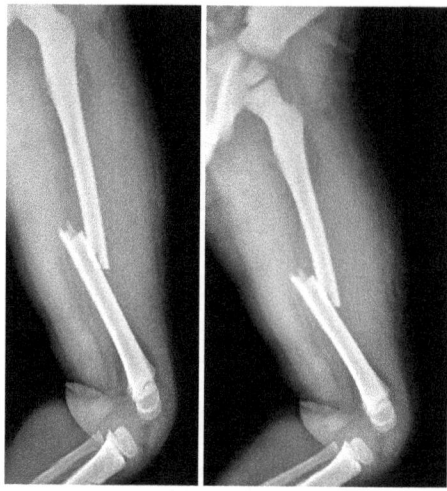

Treatment: Closed reduction and immobilization by 1½ hip spica or closed reduction and internal fixation by TENS, or by open reduction and internal fixation (ORIF) with narrow limited contact dynamic compression plate (LCDCP) with screws.

X-RAY OF FRACTURE BOTH BONE M/3 OF FOREARM IN ADULT

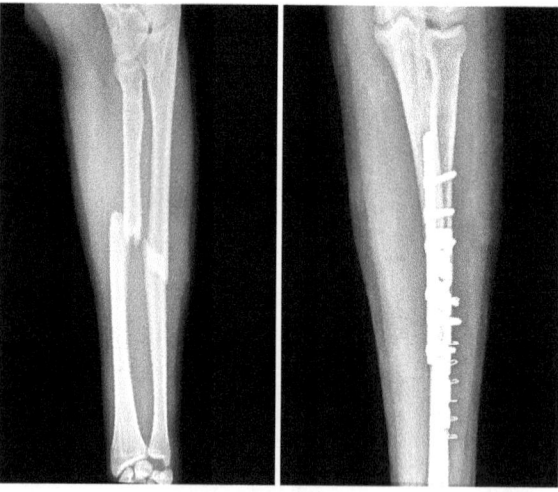

Treatment: By ORIF with limited contact dynamic compression plate (LCDCP) with cortical screws.

X-RAY OF FRACTURE BOTH BONE LEG AT M/3 AND D/3 JUNCTION

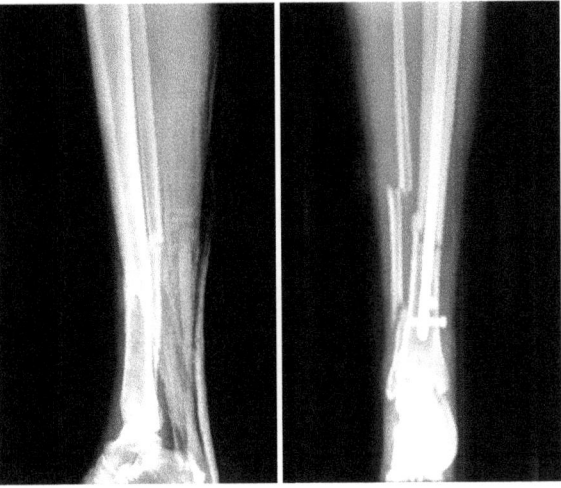

Treatment: By closed reduction and internal fixation by interlocking nail.

X-RAY OF COMMINUTED FRACTURE SHAFT OF DISTAL HUMERUS

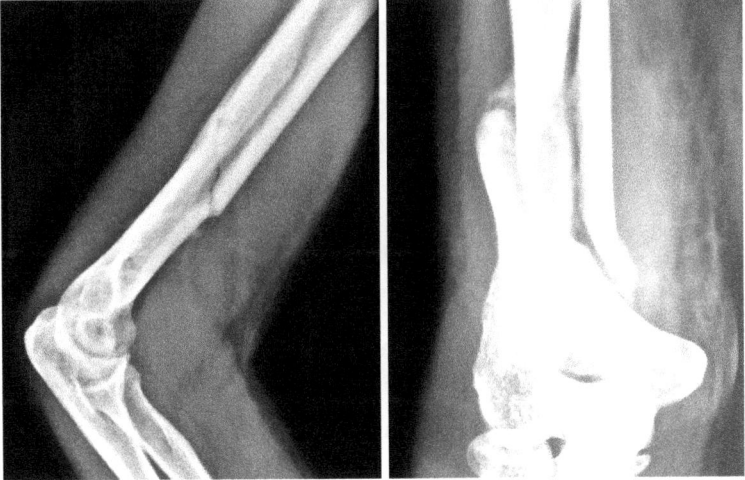

Treatment: By closed reduction and internal fixation with limited contact dynamic compression plate with screws.

X-RAY OF M/3 FRACTURE CLAVICLE

Treatment: By closed reduction and 'Figure of 8' bandage or by clavicular brace with arm sling or ORIF with clavicular plate or reconstruction plate and screws.

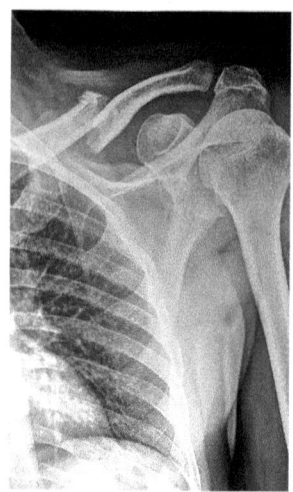

X-RAY OF FRACTURE PROXIMAL HUMERUS

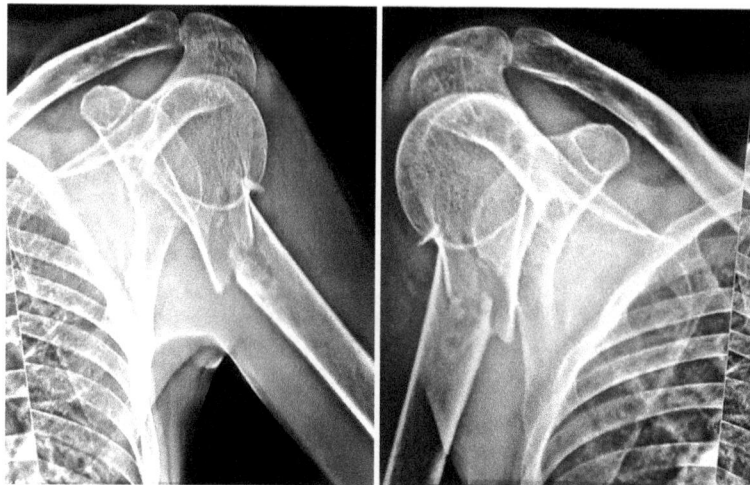

Treatment: By closed reduction and internal fixation by PHILOS plate (proximal humerus locking plate) with locking screws under image intensifier guidance.

X-RAY OF FRACTURE BOTH BONE FOREARM AT M/3 TO D/3 JUNCTION

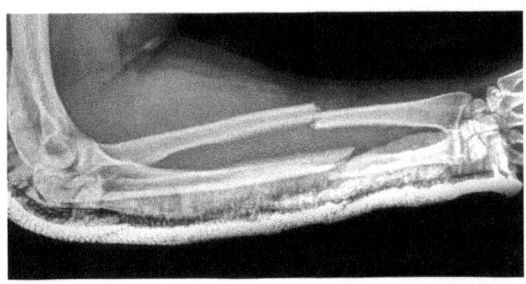

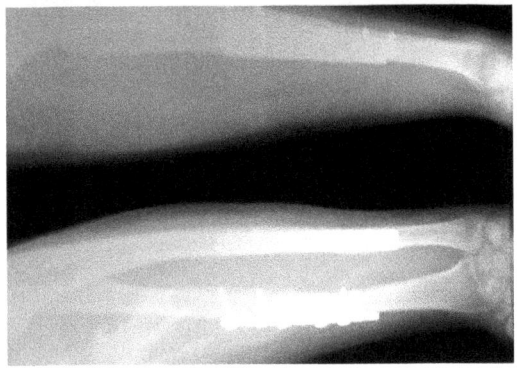

Treatment: By ORIF with LCDCP with cortical screws.

X-RAY OF FRACTURE BOTH BONE LEG (FRACTURE SHAFT OF LOWER 1/3RD OF TIBIA AND UPPER 1/3RD OF FIBULAR SHAFT)

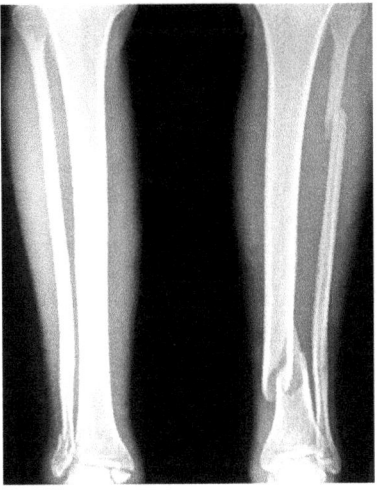

Treatment: OR + IF locking plate for fracture tibia
OR + IF 1/3 semitubular plate for fracture fibula.

INTERNAL FIXATION WITH TENS IN A FRACTURE BOTH BONE FOREARM IN CHILD AFTER CLOSED REDUCTION

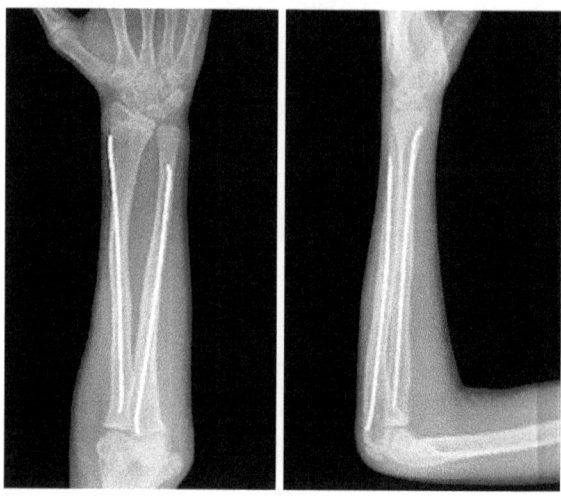

X-RAY OF FRACTURE ACETABULUM

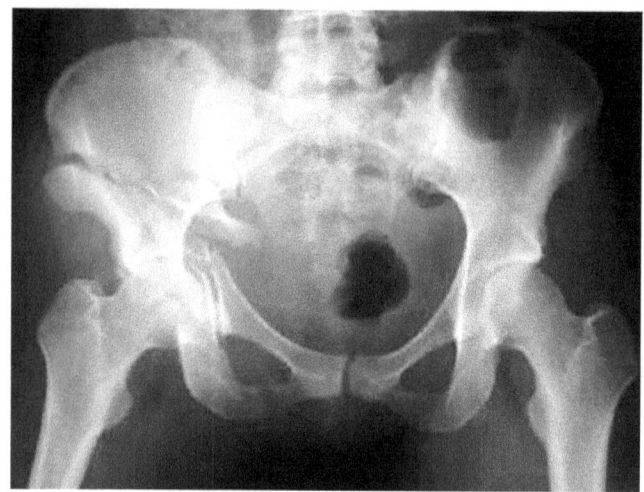

X-RAY OF FRACTURE SHAFT OF FEMUR

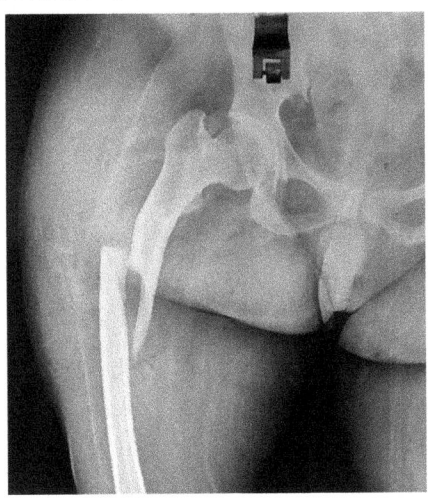

INTERNAL FIXATION WITH CLOSED INTERLOCKING NAIL WITH BOLTS IN A CASE OF FRACTURE SHAFT OF FEMUR

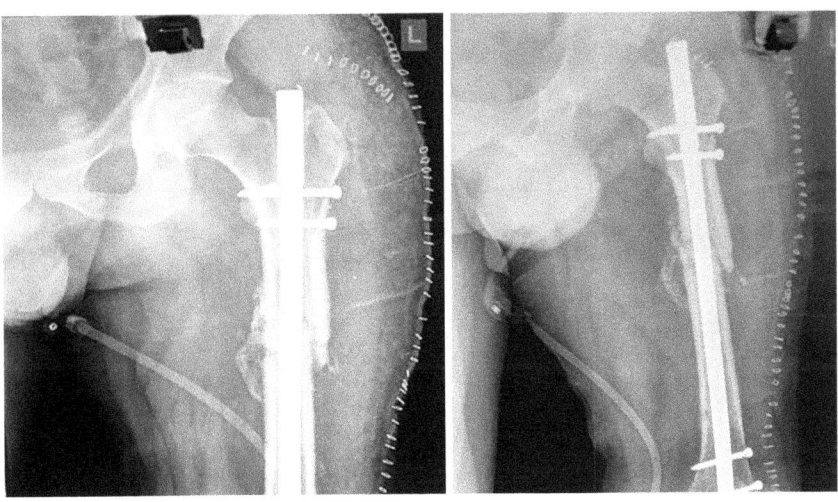

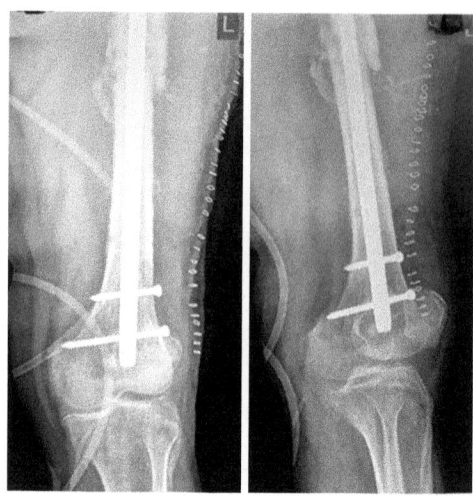

INTERNAL FIXATION WITH HERBERT (HEADLESS) SCREW FOR FRACTURE SCAPHOID, AFTER OPEN REDUCTION

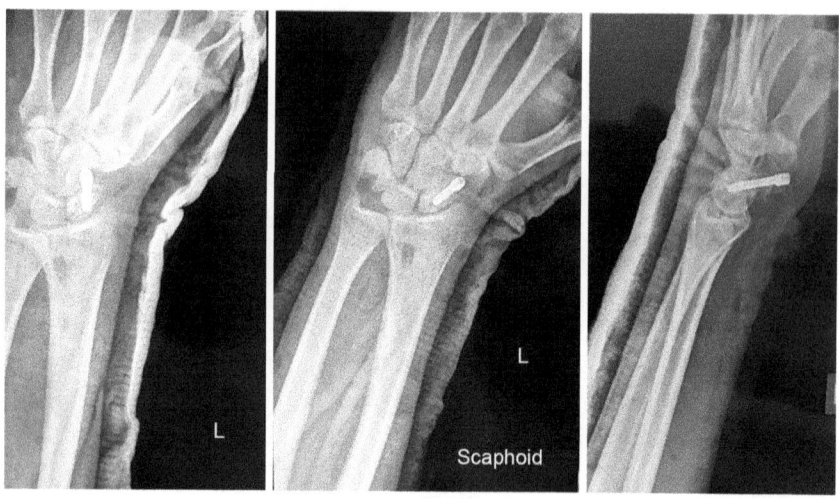

INTERNAL FIXATION WITH MEDIAL BUTTRESS PLATE AFTER CLOSED EDUCATION IN A MEDIAL CONDYLE FRACTURE TIBIA WITH K-WIRE FIXATION FOR FRACTURE NECK OF FIBULA

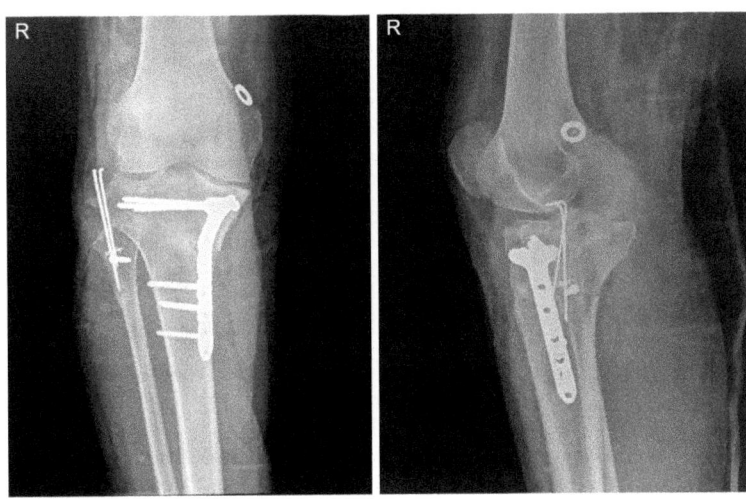

X-RAY OF FRACTURE BOTH BONE FOREAM

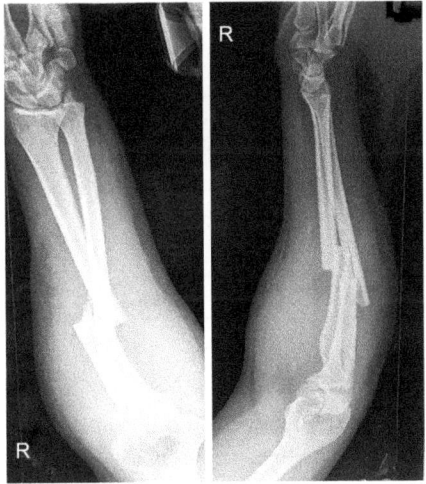

INTERNAL FIXATION WITH LCDCP FOR FRACTURE BOTH BONE FOREARM AFTER OPEN REDUCTION

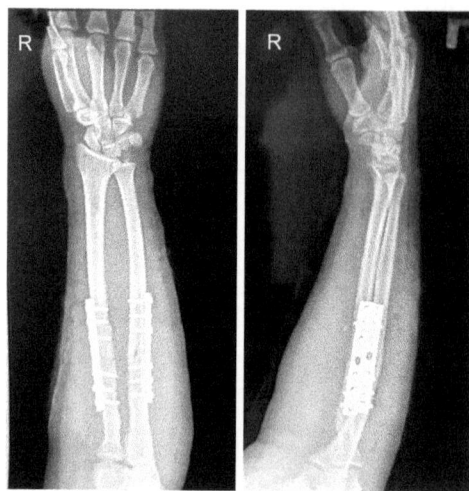

X-RAY OF FRACTURE NECK OF FEMUR

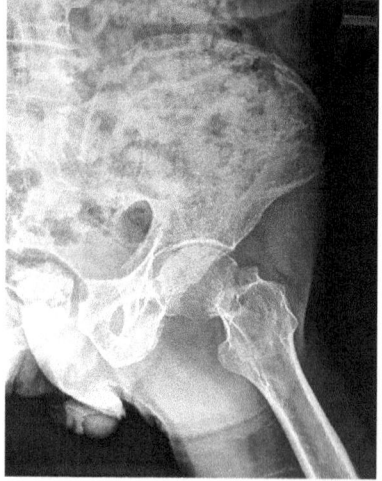

Treatment: Closed reduction and internal fixation by cannulated cancellous screw (CHS) in adult or hemiarthroplasty by Austin Moore's prosthesis (AMP) in old age.

BIPOLAR (PROSTHESIS) HEMIARTHROPLASTY IN A CASE OF FRACTURE NECK OF FEMUR, WITH AVASCULAR NECROSIS OF OPPOSITE HIP

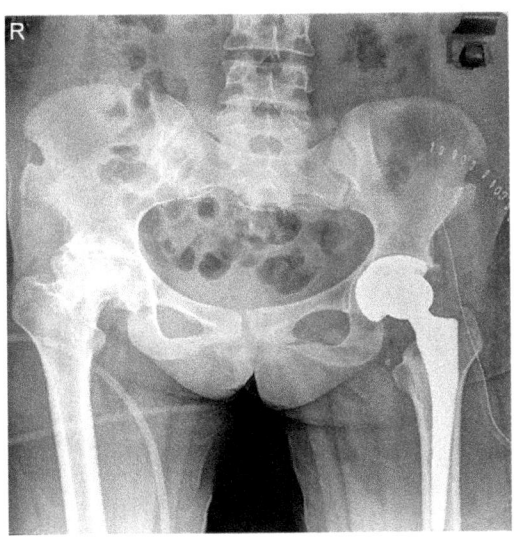

BIPOLAR (PROSTHESIS) HEMIARTHROPLASTY IN A CASE OF FRACTURE NECK OF FEMUR

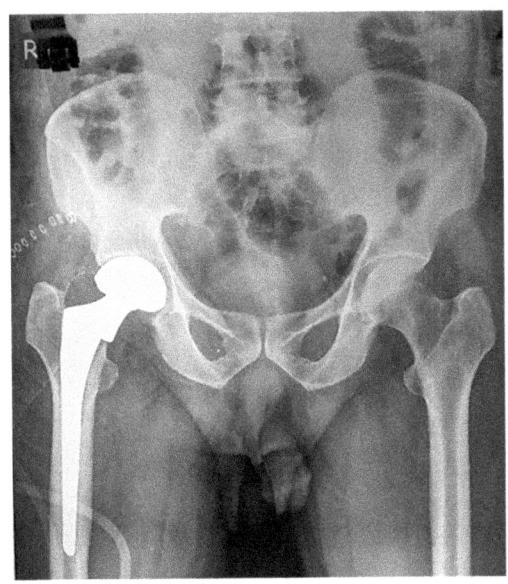

X-RAY OF FRACTURE INTERTROCHANTERIC FEMUR

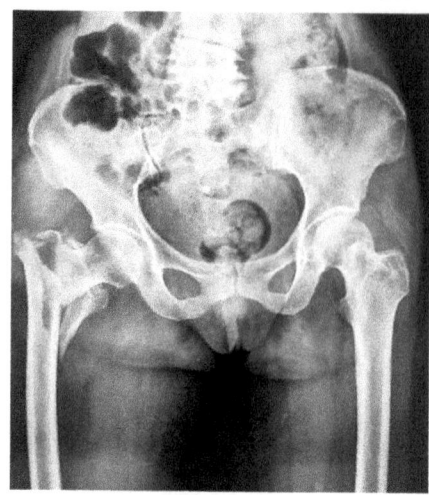

Treatment: Closed reduction and internal fixation with DHS.

INTERNAL FIXATION WITH DYNAMIC HIP SCREW WITH BARREL PLATE WITH COTICAL SCREW, AFTER CLOSED REDUCTION, IN A CASE OF INTERTROCHANTERIC FRACTURE

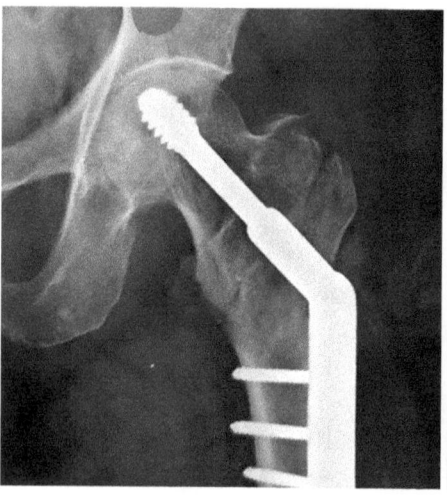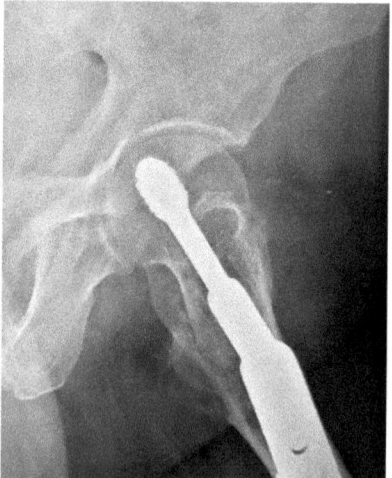

COMMUNITED FRACTURE CALCANAUM—LATERAL VIEW

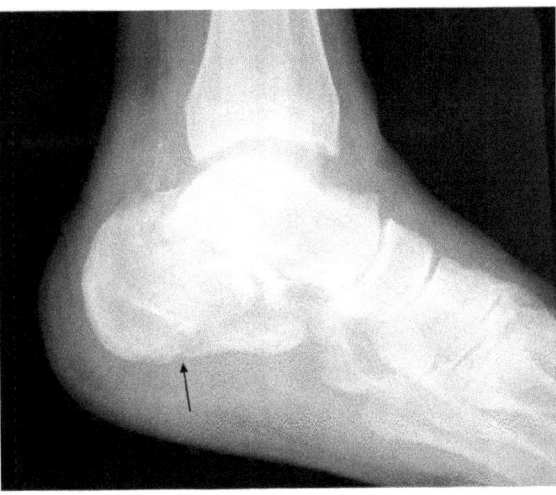

Treatment: By open reduction and internal fixation by H-plate/Y-plate or reconstruction plate.

X-RAY OF COMMINUTED FRACTURE BOTH BONE LEG

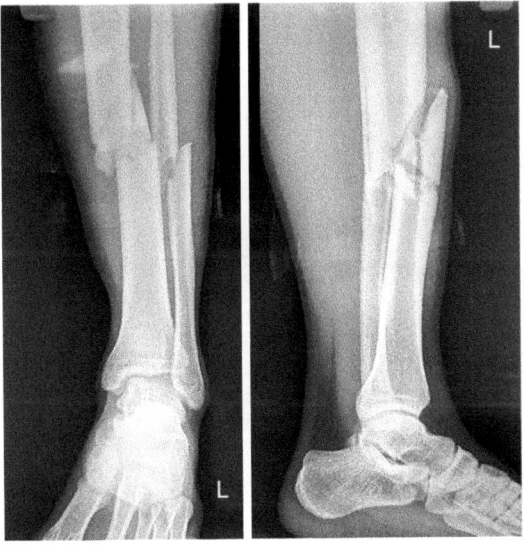

Treatment: Closed reduction and internal fixation with interlocking nail.

INTERNAL FIXATION WITH CLOSED INTERLOCKING NAIL IN A CASE OF FRACTURE BOTH BONE LEG

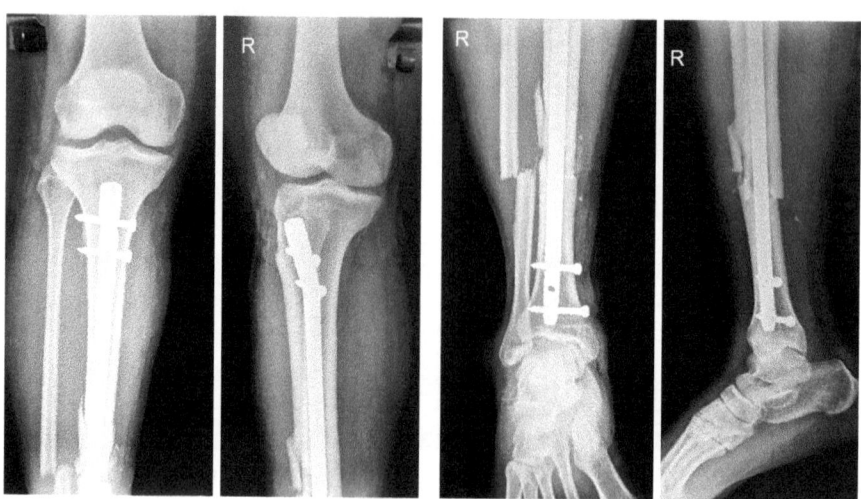

X-RAY OF UNITING FRACTURE OF BOTH BONE LEG WITH INTERLOCKING NAIL IN SITU

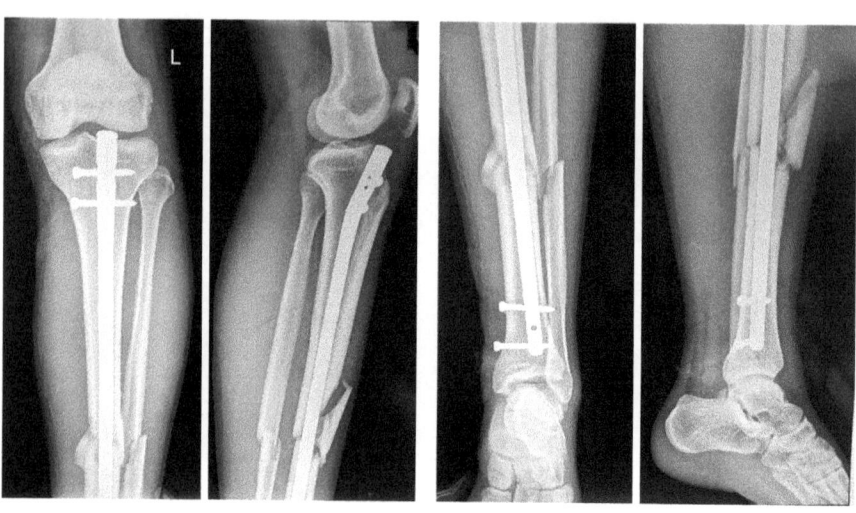

X-RAY OF FRACTURE SUPRACONDYLAR HUMERUS IN A CHILD WITH POP BACK SLAB

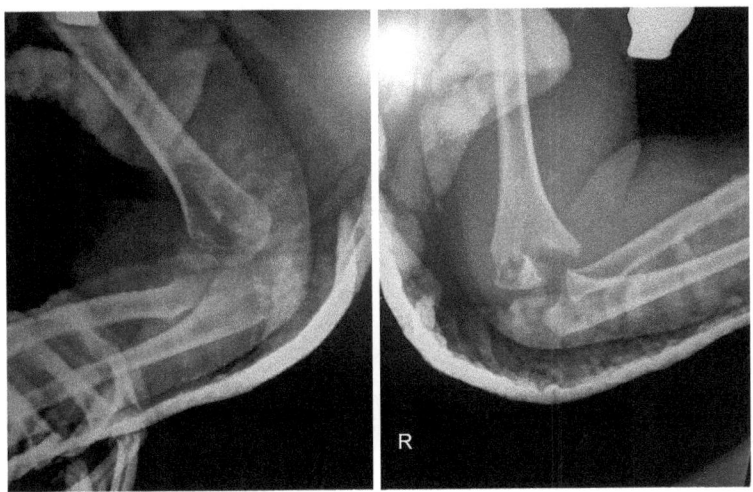

X-RAY SHOWING FRACTURE PATELLA (BOTH ANTEROPOSTERIOR AND LATRAL VIEW OF KNEE)

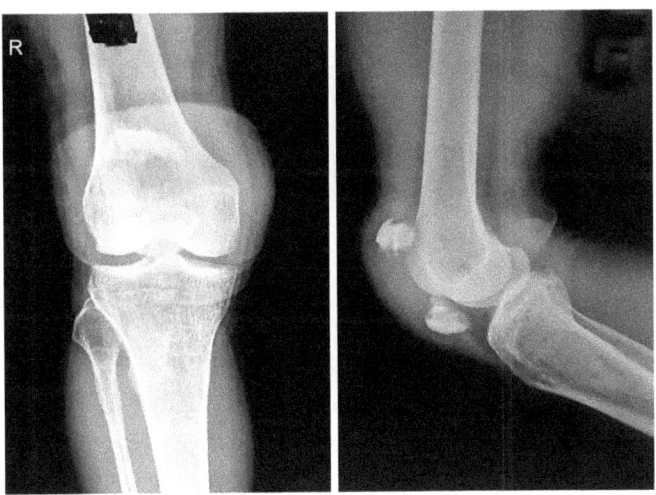

X-RAY OF FRACTURE DISTAL RADIUS (COLLES EXTRA-ARTICULAR)

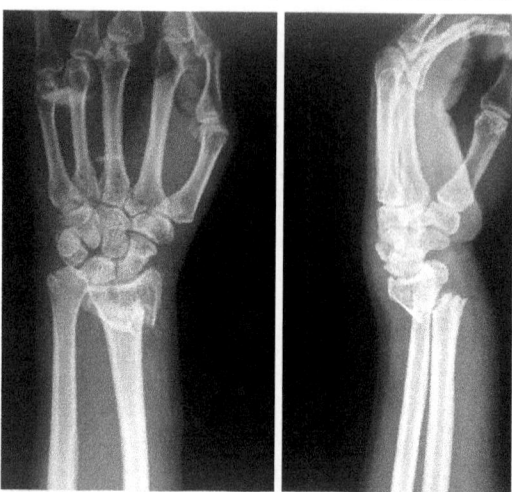

X-RAY OF GALEAZZI FRACTURE DISLOCATION (FRACTURE OF THE DISTAL RADIUS WITH DISTAL RADIOULNAR JOINT DISLOCATION)

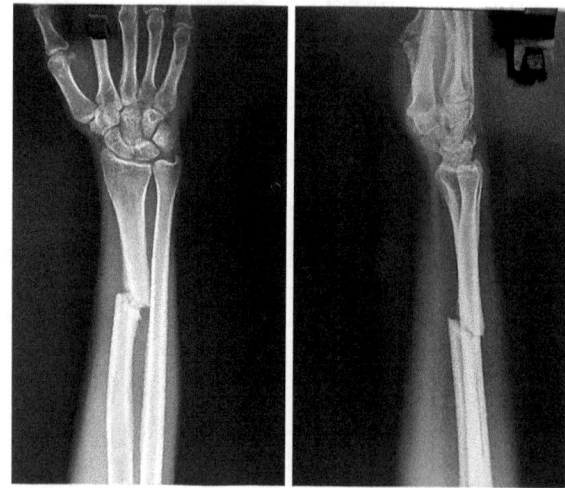

Treatment: By open reduction of the dislocated joint and internal fixation by 3.5 mm LCDCP with cotical screw.

FRACTURE NECK OF HUMERUS WITH DISLOCATION SHOULDER

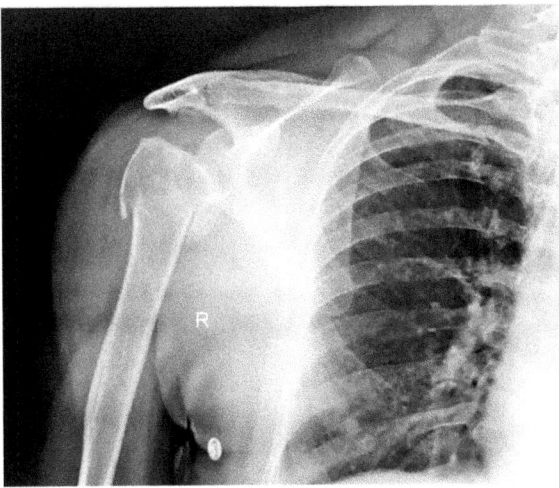

Treatment: By closed/open reduction and internal fixation by minimally invasive-plate osteosynthesis (MIPO) plate under image guidance.

X-RAY OF FRACTURE SHAFT OF HUMERUS

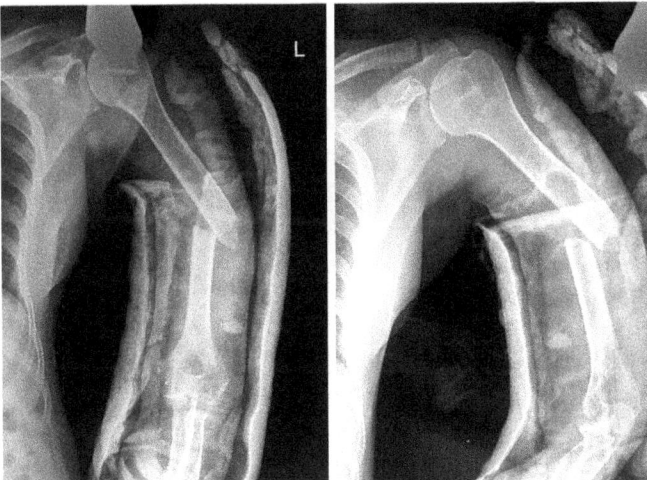

Treatment: By open reduction and internal fixation by 4.5 mm narro LCDCP or closed reduction and internal fixation by interlocking nail.

X-RAY OF FRACTURE SHAFT OF TIBIA WITH BIMALLEOLAR FRACTURE

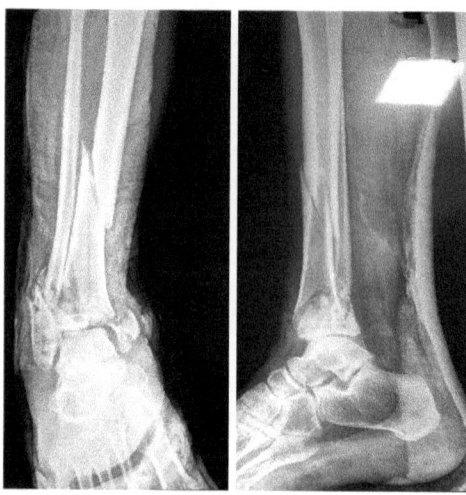

X-RAY OF DEPRESSED FRACTURE LATRAL CONDYLE OF TIBIA

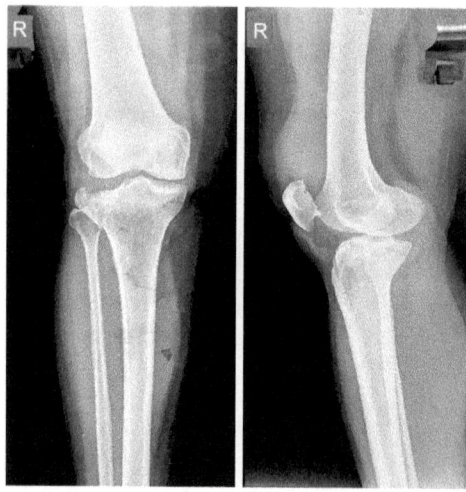

Treatment: By closed reduction and elevation of depressed fracture under imge guidance and internal fixation by lateral buttress plate.

X-RAY OF FRACTURE DISTAL RADIUS WITH VERTICAL SPLIT UP TO SHAFT

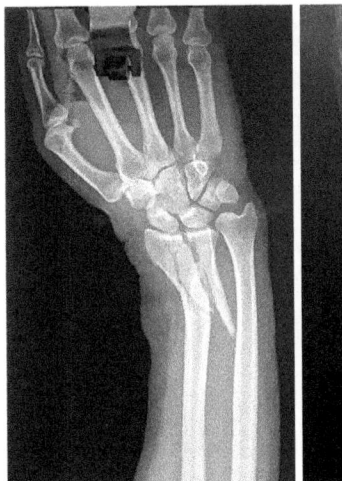
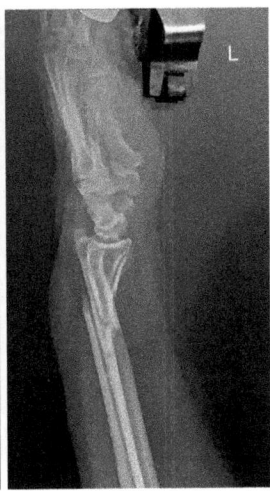

X-RAY OF FRACTURE OLECRANON

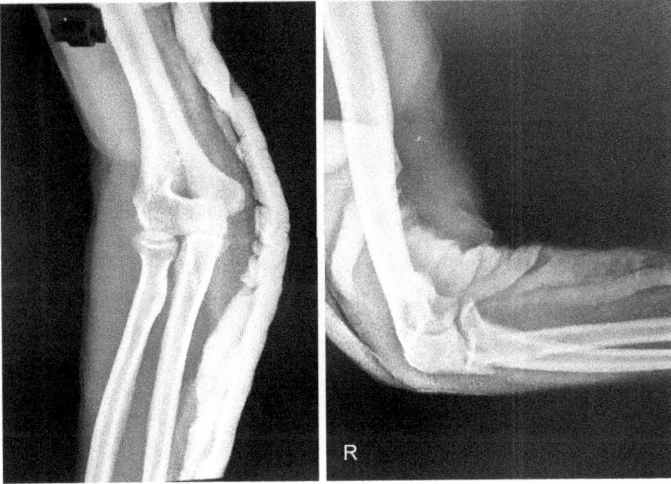

Treatment: By open reduction and internal fixation by tension band wiring.

X-RAY ANEURYSMAL BONE CYST IN LOWER END OF TIBIA

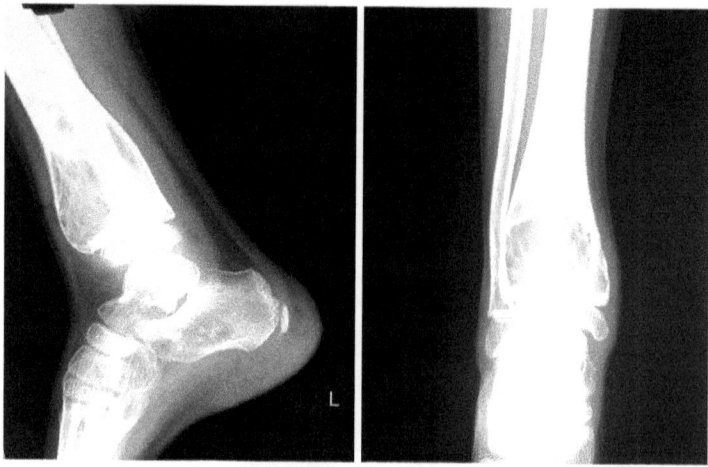

Treatment: After confirmation of diagnosis—by curettage and bone cementing.

X-RAY OF LEG OF A CASE OF OSTEOGENESIS IMPERFECTA IN A CHILD

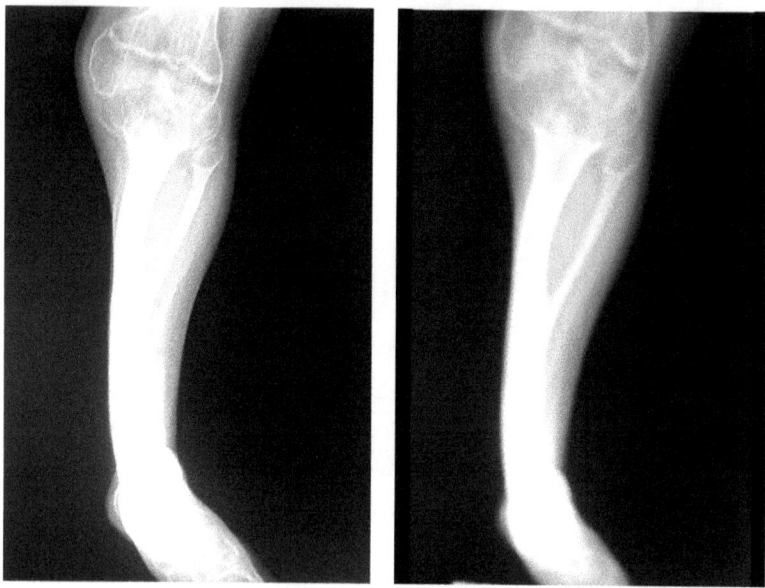

Treatment: Corrective osteotomy and internal fixation.

X-RAY OF BOTH BONE LEG IN A CASE OF OSTEOGENESIS IMPERFECTA

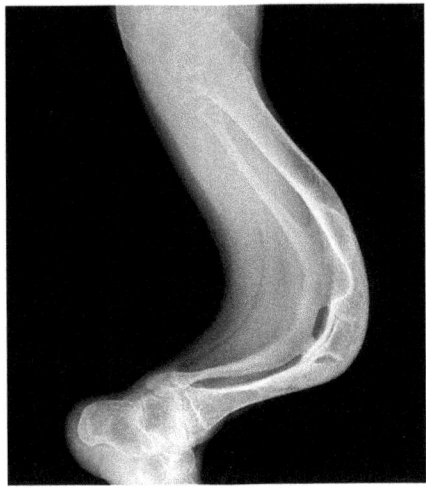

Treatment: Corrective osteotomy and internal fixation.

X-RAY OF A POST-SEPTIC SEQUELAE OF HIP

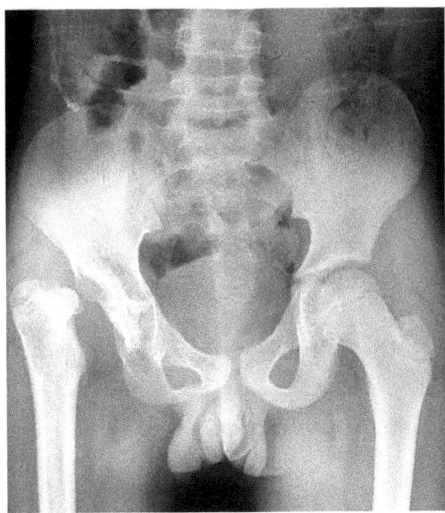

Treatment: Corrective osteotomy.

X-RAY OF CHRONIC OSTEOMYELITIS OF RADIUS IN A CHILD

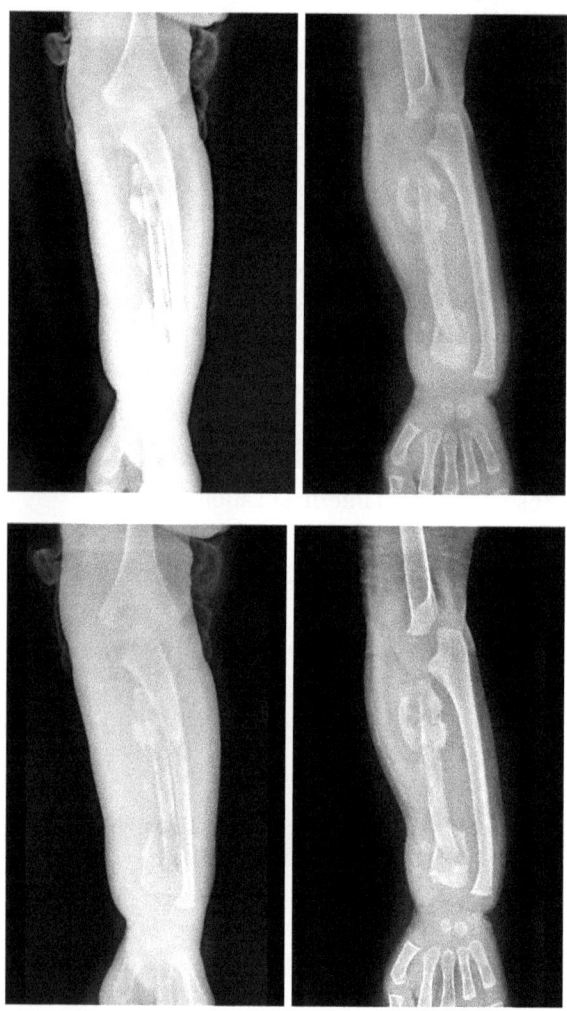

Treatment: Debridement + Curettage + Saucerization.

INDEX

A

Achondroplasia 10
Acute respiratory distress syndrome 65
Adriamycin 42
Adult hypophosphatemic rickets 33
Affected hip
    clinical examination of 108
    movement of 106, 109
Allis tissue forceps 132
Amputation 43
    indications of 44
Aneurysmal bone cyst 37, 117
    clinical features 37
    investigation 37
    X-ray 170
Ankle, examination of 107
Ankylosing spondylitis 21
    treatment of 22
Ankylosis 95
    clinical features 96
    etiology 96
    investigation 96
    treatment 96
    types 95
Antirheumatic drugs, disease-modifying 20
Antistreptolysin O 20
Arterial insufficiency 28
Arthritis 22
Arthroscopy 101
    complication 101
    technique 101
    use 101
Arthrotomy 18
Atrial septal defect 126
Austin Moore's prosthesis 141, 160
Autogenous graft, sites for 97
Avascular necrosis 28
    causes of 28
    classification of 29
    treat 29

B

Baker's cyst 100
    clinical fractures 100
    treatment 101
Below-knee amputations 44
Bholer's stirrup 142
Bimalleolar fracture 168
Bipolar hemiarthroplasty 161
Bipolar prosthesis 141
Blood 113
    biochemistry 32
Bone
    awl with hole 138
    chisel 129
    curette 133
    cutting forceps 130
    forearm 126
    gouge 133
    graft 97
    holding forceps 134, 138
    lever 131
    nibbler 131
    pliers 128
    scan 100
    tap 130
Bone leg
    uniting fracture of 164
    X-ray of 171
Bone tumors 35, 39, 51, 94
    benign 35
    malignant 35
Bony ankylosis 96
Boyd classification 57
Brodie's abscess 92
    clinical features 92
    treatment 92

C

Calcaneal wedge osteotomy 5
Cancellous schanzpin 147, 148
Cancellous screw 142
Cannulated rimmer 135
Caries spine 105, 115
Carpal tunnel syndrome 94
Cartilage capped exostosis 94
Cartilage destruction, progressive 25
Cartilage origin, bone tumorsof 94
Cervical spine, X-ray of 116
Cervical spondylosis 90
    clinical features 90
    investigation 90
    treatment 90
Chondroblastoma 94
Chondroma 94
Chondromyxoid fibroma 94
Chondrosarcoma 39, 41, 94
    clinical features 41
    pathology 41
    treatment 41
Chronic arthritis, juvenile 22
Chronic osteomyelitis 16, 92, 105, 112, 117, 172
    clinical features of 16
Cobb's angle 90
Codmann's triangle 99
    etiopathogenesis 99
    investigation 100
    treatment 100
Collateral injury
    lateral 47
    medial 47
Colles' fracture 72, 86
    clinical features 86
    complication of 86
    investigation 86
    treatment 86

Comminuted fracture
   bone leg, X-ray of 163
   calcanaum 163
Compartment syndrome 77
Congenital talipes equinovarus 1, 117
Congenital tibial pseudoarthrosis 12
Congenital vertical talus 6
Conjunctivitis 22
Cortical Schanz pin 147, 148
   with universal clamp 148
Cortical screw 142
Coxamagna 115
C-reactive protein 96
Crohn's disease 22
Cruciate ligament tear, anterior 46
Crystal deposition disorder 23
Cubitus valgus 83, 117, 120
   etiology of 83
   investigation 83
   signs 83
   symptom 83
   treatment 83
Cubitus varus 83, 117, 119
   etiology of 83
   investigation 83
   signs 83
   symptom 83
   treatment 83
Cyclophosphamide 40

D

Damage cartilages 27
De Quervain's disease 95
   clinical features 95
   etiology 95
   investigation 95
   treatment 95
Diaphyseal aclasis 9, 10
   pathology of 9
Digital Bryant's triangle 106
Dilwyn Evan's procedure 5
Dislocation of elbow 80
   clinical features 80
   complication of 80
   treatment 80
Dislocation of shoulder 73, 167
   classification of 73
   clinical features of 73
   complication 74
   investigation of 73
   treatment of 73
   types 73
Distal femoral locking plate 145
Distal femur, X-ray of fracture shaft of 151
Distal humerus, comminuted fracture shaft of 153
Distal radioulnar joint dislocation 166
Distal radius, fracture of 166
Dorsolateral spine, magnetic resonance imaging of 116
Drill bit 136
Drill guide 136
Dwarfism 10
Dwyer's osteotomy 5
Dynamic compression plate 66
Dynamic hip screw 162
   with barrel plate 145
Dysplasia hip, developmental 7

E

Ear pinna 23
Elbow
   dislocation of 80
   plain X-ray of 102
   replacement 51
Endocrine disorder 30
Eosinophilic granuloma 37
   clinical features 37
   treatment 38
Equinus 2
Erythrocyte sedimentation rate 96
Ewing's sarcoma 39, 41, 117
   clinical features 41
   treatment 41
Exostosis 35
External fixation 52
   spanner wrench for 139
   types 53

F

Familial hypophosphatemic rickets 33
Febuxostat 24
Femoral head, avascular necrosis of 28
Femur
   Fracture
      head of 58
      neck of 54, 161
      shaft of 65, 125, 126, 157
   nonunion fracture neck of 107
   postoperative X-ray of fracture shaft of 125
   preoperative X-ray of fracture shaft of 125
   shortening of neck of 115
   X-ray of fracture
      neck of 160
      shaft of 152, 157
Fibrous ankylosis 96
Fibula, fracture neck of 159
Fixed flexion deformity 108
Foot
   deformity of 20
   drop 117, 121
Forefoot adduction 2
Fore-quarter amputation 43
Fracture 50, 164
   acetabular 59
   around ankle above 61, 67
   around hip joint 54
   around knee, complication of 64
   around shoulder 72
   around wrist 86
   bone leg, X-ray of 150, 153, 155
   displaced 61
   intertrochanteric femur, X-ray of 162
   malunion of 117
   metatarsal bones 71
   phalanx 71
   plate fixation in 126
   proximal humerus, X-ray of 154
   radial head 81
   tarsal bones 70
   undisplaced 61
   unstable 60
Fracture acetabulum 59
   X-ray of 156

Index

Fracture around elbow
   joint 76
   types of 76
Fracture bone forearm 84
   clinical features 84
   treatment 84
   X-ray of 155, 159
Fracture both bone
   classification of 67
   clinical features of 67
   treatment of 67
Fracture calcaneum 70
   clinical features of 70
   mechanism of injury of 70
   treatment of 70
Fracture clavicle 72
   clinical features 72
   complication 73
   investigation 72
   treatment 73
Fracture distal
   humerus 72
   radius, X-ray of 166, 169
Fracture femoral condyle 62
   clinical feature of 62
   treatment of 62
Fracture head of femur
   complication of 59
   treatment of 59
Fracture lateral condyle of humerus
   clinical features of 79
   investigation of 79
   treatment of 79
Fracture lateral
   condyle, X-ray of 120
   malleoli 68
Fracture medial
   condyle 72
   malleoli 68
Fracture metacarpals 87
   clinical features 87
   investigation 87
   treatment 87
Fracture neck of humerus 74
   classification of 75
   clinical features 74
   treatment 75
Fracture olecranon 76, 82
   clinical features 82
   investigation 82
   treatment 82
   X-ray of 169
Fracture patella 61, 165
   clinical features of 61
   treatment of 61
Fracture pelvis 59
   treatment of 60
   X-ray of 151
Fracture phalanges 87
   clinical features 87
   investigation 87
   treatment 87
Fracture scaphoid 87
   Herbert screw for 158
Fracture shaft of femur
   clinical features of 65
   mechanism of injury of 65
   treatment of 65
Fracture shaft of humerus 75
   clinical features 75
   treatment 75
Fracture supracondylar humerus 72, 77
   complication of 78
   X-ray of 150, 165
Fracture talus 69
   clinical features treatment of 69
   treatment of 69
Frozen shoulder 96
   clinical features 97
   etiology 96
   investigation 97
   treatment 97

G

Gait 107
Galeazzi fracture dislocation 72, 85
   clinical features 85
   investigation 85
   treatment 85
   X-ray of 166
Ganglion 104
   clinical features 104
   etiology 104
   treatment 104
Garden's classification 55
Genetic disorders 1
Genu valgum 26, 117, 124
   treatment in 26
Genu varum 26, 117, 123
   reverse of 26
Giant cell tumor 38, 117
   clinical features 38
   malignant 39
   sign 39
   treatment 39
Golfer's elbow 103
   clinical features 103
   etiology 103
   investigation 103
   pathology 103
   treatment 103
Gout
   clinical features of 24
   pathology of 23
Gouty arthritis
   differential diagnosis of 24
   investigate 24
   treatment of 24
Greater trochanter 108
Green stick fracture 53
   clinical features 53
   treatment 53
Griffin's classification 57
Gustilo-Anderson classification 67

H

Haemophilus influenzae 15
Hammer 134
Hand, deformity of 20
Hemarthrosis 46
Hemostatic forceps 133
Hereditary multiple exostosis 9

Hip 105
    examination of 107
    joint capsule 29
    neglected dislocation of 105, 110
    post-septic sequelaeof 105, 171
    septic arthritis of 17, 18
Housemaid's knee 100
    clinical features 100
    treatment 100
Humerus fracture
    intercondylar of 76, 82
    lateral condyle of 79
    medial condyle 76
    neck of 74, 167
    shaft of 75, 167
Hydrocephalus 13
Hydroxychloroquine 20
Hyperparathyroidism 33
    clinical features 33
    investigation 33
    treatment 33
Hypochondroplasia 10
Hypophosphatemic rickets 33

I

Ideal amputation stump 43
    types 43
Iliac spine
    anterior superior 106
    posterior superior 106
Ilizarov's external fixator 6
Implants 141
Infection 14
Injury, mechanism of 72, 74-76, 78-82, 87, 98
Intercondylar fracture 82
    clinical features 82
    investigation 82
    treatment 83
Interlocking nail 118
    closed 157, 164
    in situ 164
Internal fixation 156-160, 162, 164
Interphalangeal joints 20
Intertrochanteric fracture 56, 162
    classification of 56
    treatment of 56
Intra-articular
    distal humerus 72
    fragments 61
Investigate rickets 32
Involucrum 16
Ipsilateral knee, examination of 107

J

Joshi's external stabilizing system 5

K

K-nail 125, 143
    with rimmer 149
Knee
    anteroposterior view of 165
    dislocation 64
    examination of 107
    lateral view of 165
    osteoarthritis of 64
Knee injury 46
    mechanism of 46
    signs 46
    symptoms 46
Knee ligament injuries 48
    clinical features 48
    investigation 49
    mechanism of 48
    treatment 49
Knock knee 26
Koch's spine 105
Kothari's angle 106
K-wire 71, 144
Kyphoscoliosis 88
    clinical features 89
    investigation 89
    treatment 90
    types 88

L

Langenbeck'sretractor 137
Lateral condyle fracture 79
    clinical features 79
    humerus 76
    investigation 80
Leflunamide 20
Leg, X-ray of 170
Ligament release 4
Limb, splintage of 66
Limited contact dynamic compression plate 118, 122, 126, 143
Locking compression plate 51
Long bone fracture
    malunion of 117
    nonunion of 117
Lower limb amputation 43
    types of 43
Lowmann's bone holding clamp 139

M

Made lung's deformity 93
    clinical features 93
    etiology 93
    investigation 93
    treatment 93
Mallet finger 98
    clinical features 98
    etiopathogenesis 98
    investigation 99
    treatment 99
Marble bone disease 11
McMurray's test 47, 48
Medial condyle fracture 78
    clinical features 78
    investigation 78
    treatment 78
Meniscal injury 47, 48
Metabolic disorder 30
Metastasis 51
Metatarsectomy 5
Metatarsophalangeal joints 20, 23
Methotrexate 20, 40, 42
Midfoot varus 2
Monteggia fracture dislocation 72, 84
Multiple epiphyseal dysplasia 11
Multiple myeloma 39, 42
    clinical features 42
    treatment 42
Myositis ossificans 102
    classification 103

Index

clinical features 102
etiology 102
investigation 103
treatment 103

N

Narathvascular sign 106
Neck of femur
　classification of 54
　clinical features of 54
　treatment fracture of 54
Needle holder 132
Neer's classification 75
Nerve conduction velocity study 102
Neurological dysfunction 13
Nonsteroidal anti-inflammatory drugs 15, 20, 42, 100, 103
Nonunion 118
　fracture 105, 107

O

Olecranon bursae 23
Open fracture 52, 67
　classify and investigation of 52
Open reduction plus internal fixation 118, 119, 122
Osteoarthritis 25
　clinical features of 26
　pathology of 25
　types 25
Osteochondroma 35, 94, 117
　clinical features of 35
　investigation and treatment of 35
　pathology of 35
Osteoclysis 118
Osteogenesis imperfecta 8, 9, 51, 170, 171
Osteomyelitis 14
　acute 14, 15, 51
　chronic 51
　clinical features 14
　pathology of
　　acute 15
　　chronic 16
　signs 14
　symptoms 14
　types 14
Osteonecrosis 28
Osteopetrosis 11, 12
Osteophytes, removal of 27
Osteoporosis 51, 30
　clinical features of 30
　preventive measures of 30
　treatment of 30
　type of 30
Osteosarcoma 39, 117
　treatment of 40
Osteotome 134

P

Patella holding forceps 137
Patellar tendon graft 49
Pathological fracture 51
　clinical features 51
　treatment 51
Pathological hip, local examination of 106
Pauel's classification 55
Periosteal chondroma 94
Periosteum elevator 128

Perthes disease 105, 113
　pathophysiology of 115
　treatment of 115
Philosplate 144
Plaster of Paris 51, 53
　cast 3
Plate fixation 126
Plate holding forceps 138
Post-septic sequelae 105, 111, 171
Prosthesis 161
Proximal femoral nail 58
Proximal focal femoral deficiency 12
Psoriatic arthritis 22
Purine metabolism, disorder of 23

R

Radial club hand 93
　clinical features 93
　investigation 94
　treatment 94
Radial head fracture 81
　clinical features 81
　investigation 81
　treatment 81
Radius
　chronic osteomyelitis of 172
　head of 76
Reconstruction plate 145
Recurrent dislocation of shoulder 74
　clinical features 74
　investigation 74
　treatment 74
Reiter's syndrome 22
Renal rickets 34
　clinical features 34
Renal tubular acidosis 56
Rheumatic disorders 19, 22
Rheumatoid arthritis 19, 20, 51
　clinical features of 19
　pathology of 19
Rickets 31, 124
　clinical feature of 32, 123
　etiology of 31
Rimmer 135
Ring fixator 6
　procedure 53
Ruptured tendo-Achilles 98
　clinical features 98
　investigation 98
　treatment 98
Rush nail 144

S

Salazopyrin 20
Salmonella 15
Scaphoid fracture 87
　clinical features 87
　complication 87
　investigation 87
　treatment 87
Schanzpin 147
Schatzkar classification 64
Screw driver 128
Semitendinosus tendon graft 49
Septic arthritis 18
　pathology of 17
Sequestrectomy forceps 129

Sequestrum 16
Shock, correction of 66
Shoulder
    dislocation of 73
    recurrent dislocation of 74
Sickle cell disease 15
Simple bone cyst 36, 117
    clinical features 36
    treatment 36
Skeletal dysplasia 9
    types of 9
Slipped capital femoral epiphysis 114
Slipped disk 88
    clinical features 88
    etiopathogenesis 88
    investigation 88
    treatment 88
Smith fracture 72
Smith-Peterson approach 18
Soft tissue release 4
Spina bifida 12, 13
    cystica 12
    occulta 13
    pathology of 12
Spinal disorders 88
Spine 105
    examination 107
    range of movement of 116
Spondylolisthesis 90
    clinical features 91
    investigation 91
    treatment 91
    types 90
Spondylosis, cervical 90
Sports injury 46
Staphylococcus aureus 16
Steinmann pin 141, 142
Stress fracture 50
Subtrochanteric fracture 57
    treatment of 58
Sulfasalazine 20
Supracondylar fracture humerus 76
    clinical features, of 76
    investigation 77
    mechanism of 76
    treatment 77
Syme's amputation 43, 45
Systemic corticosteroids 20

T

Talipes, meaning of 1
Talo 1st metatarsal angle 3
Talocalcaneal angle 2
Tardy ulnar nerve palsy 101
    clinical features 102
    investigation 102
    treatment 102
Tarsectomy 5
T-clamp 148
Tendo-Achilles 23, 98
    tenotomy of 4
Tendon release 4
Tennis elbow 103
    etiology 103
    investigation 103
    pathology 103
    treatment 103

Tension band wiring 62, 125
Tibia
    depressed fracture lateral condyle of 168
    fracture of 67
    lower end of 170
    X-ray of fracture shaft of 168
Tibial condyle, fracture of 63
Tibial plateau fracture 63
Tissue culture 96
Titanium elastic nail 118
    system 71
Torn ligaments 27
Total elbow replacement 20, 51
Total hip replacement 29, 51, 96
Total knee replacement 27, 51, 96
Transient synovitis 114
Trigger finger 99
    clinical features 99
    etiopathogenesis 99
    treatment 99
Trimalleolar fracture
    clinical features of 69
    treatment of 69
Trivial trauma 56
Trochanter, below lesser 58
Tuberculosis hip 105, 109
    joint 114
Tuberculosis spine 105, 115
Tube-tube clamp 148
Tubular fixator, procedure for 53

U

Ulcerative colitis 22
Ulnar claw hand 94, 101, 117, 122
    clinical features 94, 102
    investigation 102
    treatment 94, 102
Universal clamp 148
Upper limb amputation 43
    types of 43
Urethritis 22

V

Valgus deformity 64
Varus deformity 64
Vertebral body, compression of 31
Vinblastine 40
Vincristine 40, 42
Vitamin
    D 31
        deficient rickets 32
        resistant 33
    D_3 30
        dose of 34
Volkmann's ischemic contracture 104
    clinical features 104
    investigation 104
    treatment 104

W

Watson-Jones approach 29
Wrist drop 102, 117, 121
    clinical features 102
    investigation 102
    treatment 102

EU GSPR Authorised Reprsentative
Logos Europe, 9 rue Nicolas Poussin
1700, La Rochelle, France
Phone: +33 (0) 6 67 93 73 78
E-mail: contact@logoseurope.eu

www.ingramcontent.com/pod-product-compliance
Ingram Content Group UK Ltd.
Pitfield, Milton Keynes, MK11 3LW, UK
UKHW050456150426
5217IPUK00025B/1719